Thyroid Cancer - The Road From Genes to Successful Treatment

Edited by Ifigenia Kostoglou-Athanassiou

Published in London, United Kingdom

Thyroid Cancer - The Road From Genes to Successful Treatment
http://dx.doi.org/10.5772/intechopen.100924
Edited by Ifigenia Kostoglou-Athanassiou

Contributors
Thérèse Truong, Fabienne Lesueur, Mehdi Hedayati, Shabnam Heydarzadeh, Shirley Yuk-Wah Liu, Tom Chi-Man Chow, Yun Yu, Richard R.P.A. Crooijmans, Juan Pablo Nicola, Gerardo Hernán Carro, Aisyah Elliyanti, Kainickal Cessal Thommachan, Geethu Babu, Rejnish Ravikumar, Malu Rafi, Lekha Madhavan Nair, Zuzaki Sharafuddin, John Mathew, Nijo Jose, Mullangath Prakasan Aparna, Ifigenia Kostoglou-Athanassiou

First published in London, United Kingdom, 2023 by IntechOpen
IntechOpen is the global imprint of INTECHOPEN LIMITED, registered in England and Wales, registration number: 11086078, 5 Princes Gate Court, London, SW7 2QJ, United Kingdom

British Library Cataloguing-in-Publication Data
A catalogue record for this book is available from the British Library

Additional hard and PDF copies can be obtained from orders@intechopen.com

Thyroid Cancer - The Road From Genes to Successful Treatment
Edited by Ifigenia Kostoglou-Athanassiou
p. cm.
Print ISBN 978-1-80356-284-1
Online ISBN 978-1-80356-285-8
eBook (PDF) ISBN 978-1-80356-286-5

Meet the editor

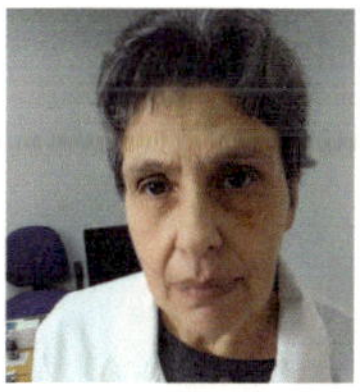

Dr. Ifigenia Kostoglou-Athanassiou is an endocrinologist who graduated from the Medical School, Aristotle University of Thessaloniki, Greece. She obtained an MD from the University of Athens Medical School and a Ph.D. from the University of London. Her areas of research include breast cancer, neuroendocrinology, melatonin, thyroid cancer, vitamin D, and autoimmune diseases. She has won several awards for her research. Dr. Kostoglou-Athanassiou has published numerous papers and book chapters. Currently, she works as a consultant endocrinologist and head of the Endocrine Department, at Asclepeion Hospital, Voula, Athens, Greece.

Contents

Preface

Thyroid cancer is the most common endocrine cancer. It is treated by thyroidectomy and radioiodine administration followed by life-long thyroxine administration. However, until recently, there was no medical treatment for advanced thyroid cancer. Advances in the genetics of thyroid cancer and in the treatment of other forms of cancer with tyrosine kinase inhibitors have enabled the application of this very recent knowledge in the treatment of advanced thyroid cancer. The application of this knowledge has revolutionized the treatment of advanced thyroid cancer.

The first section of this book focuses on the genetics of thyroid cancer. In Chapter 1, Fabienne Lesueur and Thérèse Truong discuss the genetic susceptibility to differentiated thyroid cancer. In Chapter 2, Professor Mehdi Hedayati and Dr. Shabnam Heydarzadeh examine the impact of ret-protooncogene mutations on the diagnosis, treatment, and prognosis of medullary thyroid cancer. In Chapter 3, Yun Yu and Richard Crooijmans discuss the genomics of familial thyroid cancer in dogs. In Chapter 4, Dr. Gerardo Hernán Carro and Dr. Juan Pablo Nicola review the molecular basis of radioiodine treatment in thyroid cancer.

The second section of this book focuses on treatment of thyroid cancer. In Chapter 5, Dr. Ifigenia Kostoglou-Athanassiou discusses recent developments in the medical treatment of advanced thyroid cancer. In Chapter 6, Professor Aisyah Elliyanti discusses the indications for radioiodine therapy in differentiated thyroid cancer. In Chapter 7, Dr. Thomachan Kainichal Cessal reviews systemic therapy in thyroid cancer. In Chapter 8, Dr. Thomachan Kainichal Cessal highlights recent advances in the management of anaplastic thyroid carcinoma. In Chapter 9, Dr. Tom Chi-Man Chow and Dr. Shirley Yuk-Wah Liu examine the significance of lymph node metastasis in thyroid cancer. Finally, in Chapter 10, Dr. Thomachan Kainichal Cessal discusses external beam radiotherapy in differentiated thyroid cancer.

I would like to thank the contributing authors for their excellent chapters. I also acknowledge the assistance of Author Service Manager Nika Karamatic at IntechOpen. I am extremely grateful to my family, especially my husband Dr. Panagiotis Athanassiou and my children Lambros and Yannis for their continuous help and support over the years.

Last, but not least, I dedicate this book to my mother Areti, whose example and efforts have made it possible for me to become the editor of this book.

Ifigenia Kostoglou-Athanassiou, MSc, MD, Ph.D.
Endocrinologist,
Department of Endocrinology,
Asclepeion Hospital,
Voula, Athens, Greece

Section 1

Genetics of Thyroid Cancer

Chapter 1

Genetic Susceptibility to Differentiated Thyroid Cancer

Fabienne Lesueur and Thérèse Truong

Abstract

Differentiated thyroid carcinoma (DTC) represents more than 90% of all thyroid cancer histological types. Its incidence has increased at a faster rate than most other malignancies during the last three decades and varies considerably around the world. The familial form of the disease has also become more common than previously reported, accounting for 5–15% of DTC cases. The main established risk factor of thyroid cancer is exposure to ionizing radiation, particularly if occurred during childhood. Thyroid cancer (including DTC) is also characterized by having one of the highest familial risks of any cancer supporting heritable predisposition. In spite of such a high familial risk, linkage analysis in non-syndromic DTC families (i.e. families where DTC is the primary cancer) performed two decades ago mapped several susceptibility loci but did not lead to the identification of high-penetrance causal germline variants. More recently, genome-wide association studies based on population case–control studies identified a limited number of DTC-associated loci and suggested that multiple low penetrance genes are involved in predisposition to DTC. This chapter reviews known genetic factors predisposing to DTC as well as approaches used to map them in various populations, and opens up on alternative strategies that could help to understand DTC tumorigenesis.

Keywords: differentiated thyroid cancer, familial risk, case–control study, genetic predisposition, genome-wide association study

1. Introduction

Almost 95% of patients with malignant thyroid tumors have non-medullary thyroid cancer (NMTC), which originates from follicular cells. Most NMTC are well-differentiated and include papillary thyroid carcinoma (PTC) (80–90%) and follicular thyroid carcinoma (FTC) (10–15%) while poorly differentiated thyroid carcinoma and anaplastic carcinoma are rare. C-cell-derived medullary thyroid carcinoma (MTC) are diagnosed in approximately 5% of patients [1]. Altogether differentiated thyroid carcinoma (DTC) represents more than 90% of all thyroid cancer histological types and the most frequent malignancy of the endocrine system (**Figure 1**) [2].

DTC incidence varies considerably around the world. High incidence was reported in some Pacific islands such as Hawaii, New Caledonia, and French Polynesia [3]. Ethnic differences in incidence within the same country have

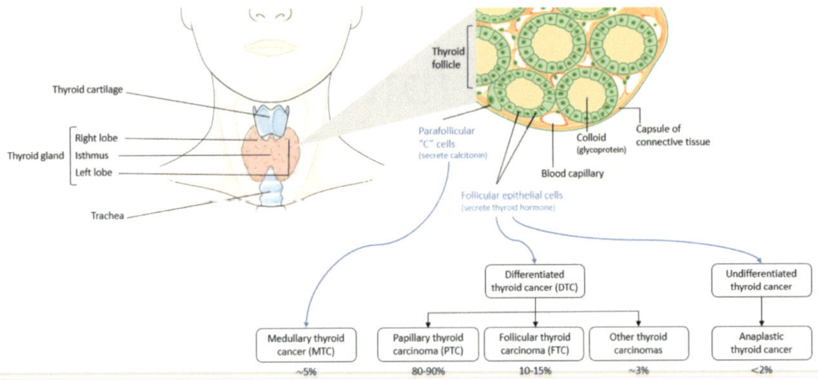

Figure 1.
Thyroid cancer subtypes classification.

been noted in Hawaii and New Caledonia with higher rates among Filipinos and Melanesians than in other ethnic groups [4]. The causes underlying these wide geographic and ethnic variations are still poorly understood. If this variation in incidence was attributed to screening practices, it was suggested that environment and inherited genetic risk factors may also play an important role [5]. Clinical awareness of potential risk factors, such as inherited genetic variants allows for earlier recognition of more vulnerable populations, earlier detection, proper treatment, and improved outcomes for patients and their families, justifying current efforts to identify and understand the causal factors and mechanisms of DTC so that effective interventions can be implemented.

Familial associations are often quantified in terms of familial relative risk (FRR). The FRR denotes the risk of disease when a family member is affected compared to the risk level in the general population. Specific types of familial relationships, like first-degree relatives, parent–child, or siblings are generally examined. Remarkably, thyroid cancer displays one of the strongest FRRs among cancers. Large case–control studies conducted in populations from Utah and Sweden showed that the FRR of thyroid cancer for first-degree relatives of probands was 8.5 and 12.4, respectively [6, 7]. Data from studies focusing on DTC conducted in Sweden, Iceland, and Norway showed that the standard incidence risk (SIR) of DTC was between 4.1 and 7.8 for male relatives and between 1.9 and 4.9 for female relatives of the proband [8–10]. The SIR for PTC was calculated in the Norwegian study as 5.8 and 4.1 for male and female relatives, respectively [10]. The family structures of non-medullary thyroid carcinoma (NMTC) patients in Taiwan were also studied. The prevalence of NMTC in the general population and in first-degree relatives of NMTC patients was 0.16% and 0.64%, respectively. This corresponds to a 5.5-fold increased risk of NMTC for first-degree family members [11].

Like many cancers, thyroid cancers may arise from mutations that may or may not be heritable. They can occur due to any mistake during DNA replication during cell division or may be induced due to the effect of carcinogens on DNA like ionizing radiation. Most thyroid cancers are the result of the accumulation of somatic mutations in the cancer genome, either driver mutations of oncogenesis or passenger mutations [12]. They are not present constitutionally in the individual but only in part of thyroid cells. By contrast, constitutional (germline) variants may predispose to cancer susceptibility and are present in affected individuals in all the body's nucleic cells, as well as the cancer genome, and may therefore be heritable. Nonetheless, over 90% of all thyroid cancers are sporadic, *i.e.* occur in people with no family history of thyroid cancer. The remaining are familial forms of NMTC and MTC. Familial MTC is associated with well-known germline genetic alterations in the *RET* proto-oncogene [13, 14] and genotype–phenotype correlations have been described [15]. On the contrary, the genetic causes of familial NMTC (FNMTC) or follicular cell-derived carcinoma are poorly understood despite considerable effort to identify contributing loci. In this chapter, we summarize variants associated with risk of DTC in familial and sporadic settings, as well as approaches used to map them in various populations and to identify causal genes or variants, which would greatly facilitate the estimation of disease risk and prognosis.

2. Familial non-medullary thyroid cancers

Familial NMTC (FNMTC) is clinically defined as the presence of the disease in two or more first-degree relatives of the patient. It encompasses a heterogeneous group of diseases, including diverse syndromic-associated tumors with a preponderance of non-thyroidal tumors and non-syndromic tumors with a preponderance of NMTC. Hereditary cancer syndromes associated with FNMTC account for 5% of all familial cases and include familial adenomatous polyposis (FAP) and its variant Gardner syndrome, Cowden syndrome, Carney complex, Werner syndrome, and DICER1 syndrome. Other syndromes with less established links to the development of NMTC include McCune-Albright syndrome, Ataxia-telangiectasia, Li-Fraumeni syndrome, and Peutz-Jeghers syndrome [16–20], also no epidemiological studies confirmed a significantly increased risk of NMTC for patients affected by these latter syndromes and for their relatives. Non-syndromic-associated conditions encompass pure familial PTC (fPTC) with or without oxyphilia, fPTC with papillary renal cell carcinoma, and fPTC with multinodular goiter [21–23]. The clinical characteristics of FNMTC are controversial. Several studies found an earlier age of onset, higher incidence of multifocality and lymph node metastasis, and a more aggressive outcome with more frequent relapses compared with sporadic disease [24], while other studies showed no significant increase in risk of recurrence or disease-related mortality in FNMTC cases compared to sporadic cases [25, 26]. Additionally, the second generation of parent-offspring FNMTC cases presents the disease at a younger age with more severe symptoms, indicating the presence of genetic anticipation [27].

Understanding the genetic basis of a heterogeneous disease such as FNMTC and the identification of biomarkers of disease aggressiveness can help to better stratify risk, allowing predictive screening of at-risk family members, improved surveillance guidance, and clinical management plan.

2.1 Genetic variants associated with risk of syndromic-associated disorders

Germline mutation (or "pathogenic variants") accounting for syndromic FNMTC are highly penetrant and actionable, meaning that targeted genet testing is recommended when the clinician recognizes the clinical phenotype of the syndrome. Clinical characteristics and genes involved in the predisposition to syndromic FNMTC are summarized hereafter.

Familial adenomatous polyposis (FAP) is inherited as an autosomal dominant trait characterized by young-onset multiple gastrointestinal adenomatous polyps, especially of the colon, with malignant potential. In about 90% of cases, FAP is caused by germline loss-of-function variants in the tumor suppressor gene *APC* (*adenomatous polyposis coli*) located on chromosome 5q21 and encoding an inhibitor of Wnt signaling pathway. Ten to 25% of germline pathogenic *APC* variants arise *de novo*. Patients with FAP or with **Gardner syndrome,** a subset of FAP in which patients also develop extra-colonic manifestations [28], have a 160-fold greater risk than unaffected individuals of developing PTC [29–31]. Two to 12% of patients with FAP develop PTC [32], and 70% to 90% of these latter are diagnosed with a cribriform-morular variant of PTC (CMV-PTC), an extremely rare variant accounting for less than 1% of all PTC in the general population [33].

Cowden syndrome (also called **PTEN-hamartoma tumor syndrome**) is an autosomal dominant disorder characterized by hamartomatous changes and epithelial tumors of the breast, thyroid, kidney, colon, and endometrium caused by germline pathogenic variants in the tumor suppressor gene *PTEN* (*Phosphatase and TENsin homolog*) on chromosome 10q23.3 in about 9% of tested probands [34]. Up to 60% of patients with Cowden syndrome have thyroid nodules and 25% of patients have thyroid cancer [35]. These patients develop principally PTC (55.1%), followed by follicular variants of PTC (19.5%) and FTC (10%) [35]. Germline pathogenic variants in genes *SDHB*, *SDHC,* and *SDHD* encoding the subunits of the succinate dehydrogenase have also been described, as well as an epimutation in the promoter of the *killin* (*KLLN*) gene [35]. Succinate dehydrogenase belongs to mitochondrial complex II that participates in both the electron transport chain and Krebs cycle, and *KLLN* is a p53-regulated gene located upstream of *PTEN* and sharing a bidirectional promoter region.

Carney complex is a dominantly inherited syndrome characterized by a classic triad of spotty skin pigmentation, endocrine overactivity, and myxomas. About 5% of patients develop thyroid nodules (follicular adenoma) and cancer (PTC or FTC). Inactivating pathogenic variants in the *PRKAR1A* gene located at 17q22–24 are identified in 73% of patients and their penetrance has been estimated to be 97.5% [36]. The gene encodes the protein kinase cAMP-dependent type I regulatory subunit alpha. Phosphorylation mediated by the cAMP/protein kinase A signaling pathway is involved in the regulation of metabolism, cell proliferation, differentiation, and apoptosis [37]. Remarkably, the *PRKAR1A* gene can fuse to the RET protooncogene by gene rearrangement and form the thyroid tumor-specific chimeric oncogene known as *PTC2* [38].

Werner syndrome is an autosomal recessive genetic instability and progeroid ('premature aging') syndrome associated with loss-of-function variants in the *WRN* (*Werner syndrome RecQ like helicase*) gene located at 8p11–21 [39]. The *WRN* gene encodes a member of the RecQ subfamily of DNA helicase protein. This nuclear protein is involved in important functions required for the maintenance of genome stability such as replication, transcription, DNA repair, and telomere maintenance. Patients with Werner syndrome develop features reminiscent of premature aging beginning in the second decade of life, including bilateral cataracts, graying and loss of hair, scleroderma-like skin changes, diabetes mellitus, and osteoporosis. They are also at elevated risk for common, clinically important age-dependent diseases, such as cancer and atherosclerotic cardiovascular disease, which are the most common causes of death at a median age of 54 years [40]. Sixteen percent of patients with Werner syndrome develop thyroid cancer, with FTC being the most common histological subtype, followed by PTC and anaplastic thyroid cancers [40].

DICER1 syndrome, also known as **pleuropulmonary blastoma familial tumor and dysplasia syndrome**, is a rare pediatric autosomal dominant inherited disorder that predisposes individuals to various benign and malignant tumors. It is caused by germline pathogenic variants in the *DICER1* gene located at 14q32.13. The gene encodes a member of the ribonuclease III (RNaseIII) family involved in the generation of micro-RNA (miRNAs) and modulates gene expression by interfering with mRNA function. In the thyroid, germline *DICER1* loss-of-function variants disrupt the correct timing and expression of miRNA production necessary for normal thyroid differentiation and function [41, 42]. Patients with DICER1 syndrome are at higher risk of early-onset multinodular goiter and thyroid carcinomas. In particular, in DICER1 syndrome families, carriers of a *DICER1* pathogenic variant have a 16-fold increase in risk of DTC as compared to noncarriers [43].

2.2 Genetic variants associated with risk of non-syndromic-associated disorders

Initial efforts to identify DTC susceptibility genes were conducted in the late 90s – early 2000s by conducting genome-wide linkage analysis in multigenerational families with multiple affected members, usually with attempt to replicate best hits in an independent set of smaller families. Some candidate genes within the mapped regions have been subsequently screened. To date, seven loci involved in FNMTC susceptibility have been mapped (1q21, 2q21, 8p23.1-p22, 8q24, 12p14, 14q32, 19p13.2), where the causal genes remain to be identified or confirmed in independent family sets. With the introduction of massive-parallel sequencing technologies in diagnostic and research laboratories in the 2010s, some of these regions have been more extremely screened highlighting new candidates (*AK023948* at 8q24, *SRGAP1* at 12p14, *DICER1*

Locus (name)	Family/ cases in the discovery study	Candidate gene	Replication study	Ref.	Approach
14q32 (*MNG1*)	1 French Canadian family, 18 MNG cases, 2 cases also with PTC	*DICER1*	Investigation of 37 NMTC families (88 DTC cases) indicates that only a small proportion of FNMTC is attributable to *MNG1*.	[23, 44]	Linkage analysis [44]; sequencing of *DICER1; in vitro* assays to assess expression level of miRNA in *DICER1* variant carriers [23].
19p13.2 (*TCO)*	1 French family, 9 PTC cases (atypical carcinomas and adenomas with cell oxyphilia); 1 family, 3 cases	*MYO1F*	No linkage in subsequent study involving 56 NMTC families [45]; WES in the original family identified *MYO1F* c.400G>A (p.Gly134Ser) but targeted sequencing of *MYO1F* in 192 FNMTC cases showed no evidence of association with FNMTC [46].	[45–47]	Linkage analysis [45, 47]; WES + functional assay + sequencing of *MYO1F* in extended sets of FNMTC families.

Locus (name)	Family/ cases in the discovery study	Candidate gene	Replication study	Ref.	Approach
1q21 (*fPTC1/ PRN1)*	1 family, 5 PTC cases, 2 family members with papillary renal neoplasia	*N-RAS, NTRK1, PRCC*	No replication study.	[22]	Linkage analysis
2q21 (*NMTC1)*	1 Tasmanian family, 8 PTC cases	*ACVR2, RAB6/ RALB, LRP-DIT*	Linkage confirmed in an independent set of 80 families.	[48]	Linkage analysis
8p23.1-p22 (*FTEN)*	1 Portuguese family, 5 PTC cases, 11 members with benign thyroid lesions	17 candidates excluded.	No replication study.	[49]	Linkage analysis + gene expression profiling + sequencing + LOH analysis.
8q24	1 family with PTC and melanoma	*AK023948* noncoding RNA (*TG* and *SLA* excluded)	Linkage confirmed using 25 additional PTC families (86 cases and 13 obligate carriers)	[50]	Linkage analysis + target sequencing+ gene expression analysis.
12q14	38 families, 108 PTC cases	*SRGAP1*	Association study on tag SNPs spanning the locus performed in 2 cases-control series from Ohio and Poland; biochemical assays showed that missense variants p.Gln149His and p.Arg617Cys impair the ability of SRGAP1 to inactivate CDC42.	[51]	Linkage analysis + association study + sequencing of *SRGAP1* + *in vitro* assays.
4q32	1 US family, 11 PTC cases and 2 cases with anaplastic thyroid carcinoma	(putative enhancer)	Not replicated in 38 NMTC families; rare single nucleotide variant absent in 2676 sporadic cases and 2470 controls from Poland and Ohio.	[52]	Linkage analysis + functional study
HABP2 (10q25.3)	1 family, 6 PTC cases	*HABP2*	Target sequencing of *HABP2* in probands of 12 Chinese PTC families [53]; sequencing of *HABP2* exon 13 in tumor from 217 sporadic PTC patients did not identify the variant [54].	[53, 54]	WES + investigation of the expression of HABP2 in thyroid tissue samples + functional assay on variant p.Gly534Glu [53]; target sequencing of *HABP2* exon 13 [54]

Locus (name)	Family/ cases in the discovery study	Candidate gene	Replication study	Ref.	Approach
16p13.3	1 family, 6 PTC cases	*SRRM2*	Identified variant c.1037C>T (p.Ser346Phe) not found in 138 familial PTC cases; association study involving 1170 sporadic PTC cases and 1404 controls confirmed association with PTC.	[55]	WES, then genotyping of identified variant in 138 other PTC; association study in sporadic PTC and unrelated controls; RNA-Seq to assess effect on efficiency of RNA splicing machinery.
15q23	34 Chinese families, 77 cases	*MAP2K5*	Variants c.961G>A and c.1100T>C identified in 2 families of the original Chinese study [56] not found in 33 Italian FNMTC families [57].	[56, 57]	WES + functional study [56]; targeted sequencing to search for the 2 previously described variants only [57]
19q13.33	1 family with 5 NMTC cases	*NOP53*	Variant rs78530808 (NOP53 p.Asp31His) identified in 3 of 44 additional families and absent in unaffected spouses; Functional studies showed oncogenic function but high frequency in the general population (MAF 1.8%) suggests a low-penetrant variant, possibly a modifier.	[58]	WES + targeted sequencing of candidate variants in familial cases and controls + functional assays.
22q12.1	5 NMTC families, 23 cases	Variants enrichment in MAPK/ ERK and PI3K/AKT signaling pathways	No replication study.	[59]	WGS
14q12	1 family with 10 members affected with PTC and/or melanoma + 23 NMTC families, 34 cases	*TINF2*	No replication study.	[60, 61]	WGS in the key family with PTC and melanoma + target sequencing of *TINF2* + gene expression analysis + quantification of relative telomere length in variant carriers and noncarriers.

Locus (name)	Family/ cases in the discovery study	Candidate gene	Replication study	Ref.	Approach
7q31.33	1 NMTC family, 8 cases	*POT1*	Another germline likely pathogenic variant in *POT1* already reported in a melanoma-prone family with occurrence of thyroid cancers [62]. Lack of likely pathogenic *POT1* variants in 7 FNMTC families [63].	[59, 64]	WGS + functional analysis, including quantification of relative telomere length in variant carriers and noncarriers

GWAS: genome-wide association study, LOH: loss of Heterozygosity, MAF: minor allele frequency, Ref.: reference, WES: whole-exome sequencing, WGS: whole-genome sequencing.

Table 1.
DTC susceptibility loci evidenced in family studies on non-syndromic NMTC (in chronological order of discovery).

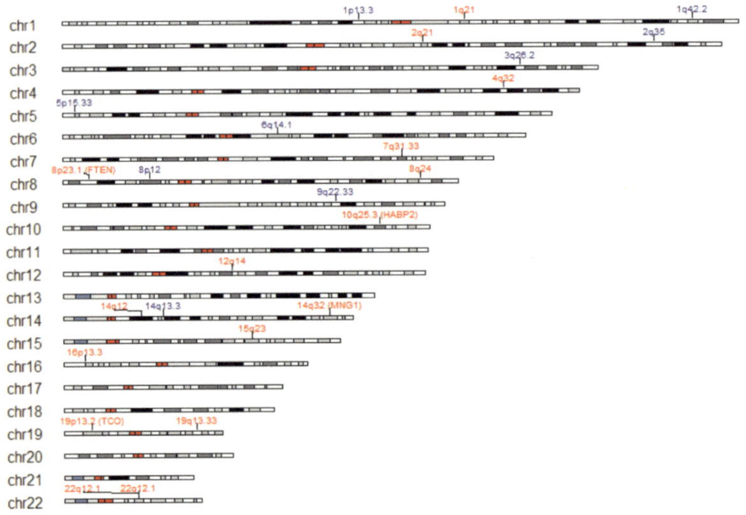

Figure 2.
DTC susceptibility loci evidenced in family studies (in red) and in genome-wide association studies (GWAS) on NMTC (in blue). Only GWAS loci replicated in independent samples are shown.

at 14q32, *MYO1F* at 19p13.2). In addition, whole-exome or whole-genome sequencing followed in most instances by functional assays allowed identification of potentially causal variants in other genes (*HABP2*, *SRRM2*, *MAP2K5*, *NOP53*, *TINF2*, *POT1*) located elsewhere in the genome. The details of these studies and clinical features of non-syndromic FNMTC families used in the discovery steps and replication steps are reported in **Table 1** and summarized in **Figure 2**.

3. Genetic factors associated with sporadic DTC

3.1 Findings from association studies

Sporadic DTC, which represents the majority of all NMTC, is considered as a complex disease caused by multiple environmental and genetic risk factors. Common polymorphisms in low-penetrance genes or altering their expression are hypoth esized to play an important role in sporadic DTC. The numerous association studies conducted in the general population used a case–control design that compares the distribution of the polymorphisms in a population of affected versus unaffected individuals. Two types of association studies can be performed: the candidate gene approach that focuses on a limited number of polymorphisms located in genes select based on *a priori* knowledge of their biological function and the genome-wide association studies (GWAS) approach that consists in screening the association between the disease and the genetic variants along the genome without prior hypothesis.

The candidate gene approach usually focuses on functional or tags polymorphisms located in specific genes selected based on their potential functional impact on the gene product or on its potential interaction with known environmental/lifestyle risk factors for the disease. Candidate genes selected for analysis in association studies on DTC are mostly involved in the following biological pathways: DNA repair, cell cycle regulation, and apoptosis, xenobiotic metabolism, thyroid function, MAPK pathway, immune response and inflammation, and obesity [65–67].

Figlioli et al. [67] proposed an exhaustive review of polymorphisms investigated in association studies published before September 2013. They reviewed 100 original articles and five meta-analyses and reported 91 significant SNPs (over 316 analyzed) from 127 genes. They also conducted a meta-analysis on 46 SNPs, which were reported by at least two studies, and reported 13 significant SNPs, of which six are located in the coding sequence of candidate genes: *ADPRT* (rs1136410; p.Val762Ala), *BRCA1* (rs16942; p.Lys1183Arg), *XRCC7* (rs7830743; p.Ile3434Thr), *TP53* (rs1042522; p.Pro72Arg), *MTHFR* (rs1801133; p.Ala222Val), *RET* (rs1800862; p.Ser836Ser), one is intronic (rs4658973 in *WDR3*) and six SNPs are located in intergenic regions highlighted by GWAS. Therefore, many candidate genes and polymorphisms were considered in association with DTC but only a few were properly replicated.

With the completion of the human genome sequencing in 2003, GWAS involving hundreds of thousands to millions of SNPs across the human genome became more and more common. GWAS are usually composed with one discovery phase that aims to analyze a large number of variants, followed by a replication phase consisting of validation of the most significant variants in an independent sample. Since 2009, seven GWAS were published on NMTC risk, of which six were conducted in individuals of European ancestry [68–73] and one was conducted in individuals of Asian ancestry from Korea [74] (**Table 2**). The latest GWAS conducted by Truong et al. [73] also included a small discovery sample of individuals of Oceanian ancestry but with no replication set. Among the GWAS conducted in the European ancestry population, one study focused on radiation-related PTC, with cases recruited in Belarus and aged 0–18 years old at the time of the Chernobyl accident [69]. All these GWAS were based on a relatively low number of cases compared to other cancers GWAS and the largest study included 3,001 cases is a meta-analysis of several studies with no replication phase [72].

Reference	Populations	Histology	Number of cases/ controls in discovery phase	Number of cases/controls in replication phase
[68]	Iceland	NMTC	192 /37,196	
	Spain	NMTC		89 /1,343
	USA (Columbus)	PTC		294/384
[69]	Belarus (Gomel) and Russia	PTC	401/620	259/648
	Age <18 years old at the time of Chernobyl accident			
[70]	Italy	PTC	701/499	
	Italy	DTC		1213/989
	Italy	DTC		326/730
	Poland	DTC		468/470
	UK	DTC		509/1,118
	Spain	DTC		443/420
[71]	Spain	DTC	398/502	
	Italy	DTC		541/532
	Spain (Galicia)	DTC		240/531
	Spain (Catalonia)	DTC		354/408
[74]	Korea	DTC	470/8,279	615/605
[72]	Iceland	NMTC	1,003/278,991	
	Netherlands	NMTC	85/4,956	
	USA (Columbus)	PTC	1,580/1,628	
	USA (Houston)	PTC	250/363	
	Spain (Zaragosa)	NMTC	83/1,612	
[73]	European descents from France, French Polynesia, New Caledonia, Belarus, Cuba	DTC	1,554/1,973	
	Oceanian from France Polynesia, New Caledonia	DTC	301/348	
	USA (Columbus)	PTC		1,580/1,628
	Italy	DTC		649/431

NMTC: non-medullary thyroid carcinoma, DTC: differentiated thyroid carcinoma, PTC: papillary thyroid carcinoma, TSH: thyroid stimulating hormone

Table 2.
Details on published genome-wide association studies on NMTC risk.

Tables 3 and **4** summarize the significant and suggestive loci highlighted by these seven GWAS. All these variants are located in intronic or intergenic regions, except rs6793295 which is a missense variant in *LRRC34* at 3q26.2. The loci that were replicated in independent studies are shown in **Figure 2**. The most robust associations, *i.e.* the ones that were reported by several GWAS and independent sample sets, are for variants at 9q22.33, 14q13.3, 2q35, and 8p12.

Locus	Nearest gene(s)	Location	Lead SNPs	EA/OA	EAF	OR	p-value	Ref.	Ancestry	Remarks	Replicated
9q22.33	FOXE1,	PTCSC2 intron	rs965513	A/G	0.34	1.75	1.7×10^{-27}	[68]	Eur		[75–89]
	PTCSC2				0.34	1.65	4.8×10^{-12}	[69]	Eur	radiation-related DTC	
					–	1.78	2.7×10^{-10}	[70]	Eur		
					0.33	1.65	2.7×10^{-23}	[71]	Eur		
		PTCSC2 intron	rs1588635	A/C	0.40	1.69	2.0×10^{-58}	[72]	Eur	r2 = 0.99 with rs965513 in EUR	
					0.39	1.64	2.1×10^{-21}	[73]	Eur		
		Intergenic	rs72753537	C/T	0.07	1.41	7.7×10^{-6}	[74]	Asian	r2 = 0.001 with rs965513 in EAS	
14q13.3	NKX2-1,	PTCSC3 promoter	rs944289	T/C	0.57	1.37	2.0×10^{-9}	[68]	Eur		[75, 79, 80, 82–84, 87–89, 92–94]
	PTCSC3			T/C	0.56	1.24	1.5×10^{-5}	[71]	Eur		
				T/C	0.46	1.25	1.4×10^{-6}	[74]	Asian		
		Intergenic	rs116909374	T/C	0.03	1.81	1.1×10^{-16}	[72]	Eur	r2 = 0.006 with rs944289 in EUR	[79, 82, 88, 93]
					0.06	2.33	1.6×10^{-10}	[73]	Eur		
		Intergenic	rs368187	G/C	0.58	1.39	5.1×10^{-23}	[72]	Eur	r2 = 0.70 with rs944289 in EUR	[93]
					0.63	1.47	3.8×10^{-13}	[73]	Eur	r2<0.01 with rs116909374 in EUR	
		Intron	rs34081947	T/C	0.41	1.27	1.2×10^{-7}	[74]	Asian	r2 = 0.61 with rs944289 in EAS r2 = 0.90 with rs368187 in EAS	

Locus	Nearest gene(s)	Location	Lead SNPs	EA/OA	EAF	OR	p-value	Ref.	Ancestry	Remarks	Replicated
2q35	DIRC3	Intron	rs6759952	T/C	0.38	1.25	6.4×10^{-10}	[70]	Eur		[108]
		Noncoding transcript	rs11693806	C/G	0.32	1.43	1.5×10^{-24}	[72]	Eur	r2 = 0.45 with rs6759952 in EUR	
		Noncoding transcript	rs3821098	T/C	0.28	1.39	1.1×10^{-10}	[73]	Eur	r2 = 0.98 with rs11693806 in EUR	
		Intron	rs12990503	G/C	0.63	1.34	3.5×10^{-9}	[74]	Asian	r2 = 0.97 with rs11693806 in EAS	
8p12	NRG1	Intron	rs2466076	G/T	0.48	1.32	1.5×10^{-17}	[72]	Eur	r2 = 0.94 with rs2439302 in EUR	
		Intron	rs142450470	T/-	0.35	1.33	1.5×10^{-7}	[73]	Eur	r2 = 0.45 with rs2439302 in EUR Significant for PTC ($p = 9.4 \times 10^{-9}$)	
		Intron	rs2439302	G/C	0.21	1.37	1.4×10^{-9}	[74]	Asian	r2 = 0.95 with rs2466076 in EAS r2 = 0.39 with rs142450470 in EAS	[73, 84, 88, 89, 92, 94, 98]
		Intron	rs6996585	G/A	0.23	1.39	1.1×10^{-10}	[74]	Asian	r2 = 0.67 with rs2439302 in EAS	
		Intron	rs12542743	C/T	0.25	1.36	4.6×10^{-10}	[74]	Asian	r2 = 0.37 with rs2439302 in EAS	

EA: effect allele, OA: other allele, EAF: effect allele frequency, lead SNP: SNP with the lowest p-value in the locus, OR: Combined odds ratio for EA versus OA from the meta-analysis of the discovery and replication sets, Ref.: Reference of the GWAS, EAS: East Asian ancestry population from the 1000 genomes project, EUR: European ancestry population from the 1000 genomes project

Table 3.
Findings from genome-wide association studies on NMTC at robust susceptibility loci (in chronological order of discovery).

Locus	Nearest gene(s)	Location	Lead SNPs	EA/OA	EAF	OR	p-value	Ref.	Ancestry	Remarks	Replicated
1q42.2	*PCNXL2*	Intron	rs12129938	A/G	0.79	1.32	4.0×10^{-11}	[72]	Eur		[109]
	PCNXL2	Intron	rs4649295	T/C	0.82	1.43	6.0×10^{-8}	[74]	Asian	r2 = 0.67 with rs12129938 in EAS	[109]
10q.24.33	*OBFC1*	Intergenic	rs7902587	T/C	0.11	1.41	5.4×10^{-11}	[72]	Eur		
5q22.1	*EPB41L4A*	Intron	rs73227498	A/T	0.87	1.37	3.0×10^{-10}	[72]	Eur		
15q22.33	*SMAD3*	Intron	rs2289261	C/G	0.68	1.23	3.1×10^{-9}	[72]	Eur		
	SMAD3	Intron	rs56062135	T/C	0.25	1.24	4.9×10^{-9}	[72]	Eur		
16q23.2	*MAF*	Intergenic	rs16950982	G/A	0.37	1.22	4.7×10^{-9}	[73]	Eur		
12q14.3	*MSRB3*	Intron	rs11175834	T/C	0.15	1.37	4.3×10^{-8}	[74]	Asian		
1p13.3	*VAV3*	Intron	rs4915076	T/C	0.70	1.33	8.5×10^{-8}	[74]	Asian		[110]
3q26.2	*LRRC34*	Exon, p.Ser249Gly	rs6793295	T/C	0.76	1.23	2.7×10^{-8}	[72]	Eur		
5p15.33	*TERT*	Intron	rs10069690	T/C	0.27	1.20	3.2×10^{-7}	[72]	Eur		[111, 112]
	TERT	Intron	rs7726159	A/C	0.39	1.17	5×10^{-6}	[73]	Eur	r^2 = 0.44 with rs10069690 in EUR	
19p12	*ZNF257*	Intron	rs7260863	T/C	0.20	1.22	8.7×10^{-7}	[73]	Eur		
4q21.1	*SEPT11*	Intergenic	rs1874564	G/A	0.69	1.31	2.0×10^{-7}	[74]	Asian		
3p14.2	*FHIT*	Intergenic	rs9858271	G/A	0.43	1.26	6.8×10^{-7}	[74]	Asian		
1p31.3	*NFIA*	Intron	rs334729	C/T	0.05	1.43	7.6×10^{-7}	[73]	Eur		
7q31.1	*IMMP2L*	Intron	rs7800391	T/C	0.34	1.25	5.7×10^{-6}	[70]	Eur	Specific to Italian pop	
	IMMP2L	Intron	rs10238549	C/T	0.63	1.27	4.1×10^{-6}	[70]	Eur	Specific to Italian pop	
3q25.32	*RARRES1*	Intron	rs7617304	A/G	0.25	1.25	4.6×10^{-5}	[70]	Eur	Specific to Italian pop	

Locus	Nearest gene(s)	Location	Lead SNPs	EA/OA	EAF	OR	p-value	Ref.	Ancestry	Remarks	Replicated
10q26.12	*WDR11-AS1*	Intron	rs1254167	C/G	0.08	1.38	5.9×10^{-5}	[71]	Eur		
	WDR11-AS1	Intron	rs10788123	T/C	0.20	1.69	3.2×10^{-5}	[71]	Eur		
9q34.3	*SNAPC4/ CARD9*	Intergenic	rs10781500	C/T	0.60	1.23	3.5×10^{-5}	[70]	Eur	Specific to Italian pop	
19p13.2	*INSR*	Intron	rs7248104	A/G	0.36	1.22	2.0×10^{-5}	[74]	Asian		
6q14.1	*HTR1B*	Intergenic	rs4075570	G/A	0.35	0.82	2.0×10^{-4}	[71]	Eur		[113]

EA: effect allele, EAF: effect allele frequency, lead SNP: SNP with the lowest p-value in the locus, OR: Combined odds ratio for EA versus OA from the meta-analysis of the discovery and replication sets, Ref.: Reference of the GWAS, EAS: East Asian populations from the 1000 genomes project, EUR: European populations from the 1000 genomes project.

Table 4.
Other significant or suggestive susceptibility loci highlighted by genome-wide association studies on DTC (ordered by significance of association).

3.1.1 Locus 9p22.33

At 9p22.33, the most robust association reported in GWAS was for rs96551 or rs1588635, a highly correlated proxy (r^2 = 0.99 in the European population from the 1000 Genomes Project). Rs965513 has been associated with radiation-related DTC as well as with sporadic DTC, and it was subsequently consistently replicated in several different populations of European ancestry [75–82], of Asian ancestry [81, 83–85] as well as in admixed populations from Oceania [79, 86], Cuba [87], Colombia [88], or Kazakhstan [89].

In 2009, a study focusing on the role of *FOXE1* in DTC risk [90] suggested rs1867277 as a causal variant at 9p22.33. This variant is located in the 5' UTR of *FOXE1* (also known as *TTF2,* for *Thyroid Transcription Factor 2*) and was shown to affect the transcription of *FOXE1* which is involved in the development and regulation of the thyroid gland, and in the proliferation and differentiation of thyroid follicular cells. However, rs1867277 is less consistently replicated in other populations and the linkage disequilibrium (LD) between rs1867277 and rs965513 is moderate in Europeans (r2 = 0.3 in Europeans from the 1000 Genomes project) and even weaker in populations of Asian or African ancestries (r^2<0.01 in the 1,000 Genomes Project). Rs965513 is located 60 kb upstream of rs1867277, in an intron of the long intergenic noncoding RNA (lincRNA) *PTCSC2* that was reported for the first time in 2015 by He et al. [91]. The risk allele [A] of rs965513 was shown to significantly decrease the expression of unspliced *PTCSC2*, FOXE1, and TSHR in normal thyroid tissue.

3.1.2 Locus 14q13.3

Rs944289 was the first variant identified by GWAS at 14q13.3 [68]. This association was replicated in subsequent studies conducted in diverse populations [75, 79, 80, 82–84, 87–89, 92–94]. However, the most recent GWAS, conducted in several European populations [72, 73] and in one Asian population from Korea [74], analyzed a higher number of SNPs (using genotyped and imputed SNPs) and reported the strongest signal for respectively rs368187 and rs34081947 (r^2 = 0.98 in Europeans and r^2 = 0.90 in East Asians from the 1000 Genomes Project), which are in moderate LD with rs944289 (r^2<0.70 in Europeans or East Asians from the 1000 Genomes Project). The recent European GWAS also reported an independent signal at rs116909374 and rs368187. Rs116909374 replicated only in studies on European ancestry populations [79, 82, 88, 93] as this SNP is monomorphic or very rare in Asian populations. Interestingly, rs368187 is in high LD with rs34081947, which was highlighted by the GWAS conducted in the Korean population (r2 = 0.98 in East Asians from the 1000 Genome Project) (**Table 3**).

In 2012, Jendrzejewski et al. [95] described a novel lincRNA named *PTCSC3* located 3.2 kb downstream of rs944289. They showed that the expression of *PTCSC3* was strongly down-regulated in thyroid tumor tissue and that the risk allele [T] of rs944289 was associated with up-regulation of *PTCSC3* in normal thyroid tissue, suggesting that *PTCSC3* could act as a tumor suppressor gene. Most recent fine-mapping analyses [79, 93] confirmed that multiple independent SNPs are involved in DTC risk at 14q13.3, but the clinical significance of all these SNPs is still unknown.

3.1.3 Locus 2q35

The association between DTC and variants at 2q35 was first highlighted in 2009 in a GWAS that investigated genetic factors associated with thyroid stimulating hormone

(TSH) levels in blood in 27,758 Icelandic individuals. The authors further investigated the role of the top SNPs associated with circulating TSH levels in DTC susceptibility of which rs966423 at 2q35 [82]. Another GWAS on DTC risk, conducted in 2013 in an Italian population [70], reported rs6759952 as the lead SNP at 2q35, which is moderately correlated to rs966423 (r^2 = 0.69 in Europeans from the 1000 Genomes project). The most recent GWAS from 2017 [72–74] reported three new SNPs (rs11693806, rs3821098, and rs12990503) with the strongest signal at 2q35, which are highly correlated to each other but only moderately with the two previous reported SNPs (**Table 2**).

Finally, the recent *in silico* fine-mapping analysis at 2q35 conducted in a multiethnic study pinpointed rs16857609 as a possible causal SNP [96]. This SNP was strongly correlated to the three SNPs reported by recent GWAS and was associated with the expression of the two nearby genes *DIRC3* and *IGFBP5* in thyroid tumor cells. Interestingly, this SNP had also been previously associated with breast cancer risk [97].

3.1.4 Locus 8p12

At 8p12, rs2439302 was first highlighted in the Icelandic GWAS on TSH levels, and it was found to be associated with DTC risk in subsequent analyses [82]. The association between DTC and rs2439302 was then replicated in different populations [84, 88, 89, 92, 94, 98]. The recent GWAS [72–74] replicated this SNP and also reported several other variants within the gene *NRG1* that were independently associated with DTC in European and Asian ancestry populations (rs142450470, rs6996585, and rs12542743) (**Table 2**).

In 2018, He et al. [99] reported that the risk allele [G] of rs2439302 was associated with the expression of multiple NGR1 isoforms in normal thyroid tissue. They also suggested that multiple enhancer variants exist at this locus that may have a combinatory effect on the expression of *NRG1* and possibly on the susceptibility to DTC.

3.1.5 Other loci

Among the other loci reported by GWAS, only SNPs at four loci (1q42.2, 5p15.33, 1p13.3, 6q14.1) were replicated in independent studies on DTC (**Table 4**). Interestingly, some of the variants reported in **Table 4** were also previously associated with other diseases or traits. For instance, the SNPs at 5p15.33 (*TERT*) were shown to be associated with telomere length in European and Asian populations [100–102] as well as with risk of breast or ovarian cancers [100, 103]. Rs7902587 at 10q24.33 (*OBFC1*) was significantly associated with ovarian cancer [104], rs56062135 (*SMAD*) at 15q22.33 was also highlighted by a GWAS on coronary artery disease [105], the missense variant rs6793295 (*LRRC34*) at 3q26.2 was associated to systemic sclerosis [106], and rs7248104 (*INSR*) at 19p13.2 was associated to triglyceride levels [107].

3.2 Polygenic risk scores

Based on findings from GWAS, polygenic risk scores (PRS), which are calculated by computing the sum of risk alleles of identified susceptibility SNPs weighted by the effect size estimate from the GWAS, were proposed to predict DTC risk. Several studies evaluated a DTC PRS in different populations [114–118]. The most recent studies used PRS including 10 to 12 SNPs reported by the meta-analysis of GWAS [72] and estimated odds ratios per standard deviation of PRS from 1.55 to 2.31. Liyanarachchi et al. [118] estimated that about 8% of the genetic predisposition to PTC could be accounted for by 10 SNPs (rs12129938, rs11693806, rs6793295, rs73227498, rs2466076, rs1588635, rs7902587, rs368187, rs116909374, rs2289261). They also estimated that individuals of European ancestry in the highest decile of PRS had a 6.9 higher risk to develop PTC than individuals in the lowest decile group. A recent study reported that the PRS improved significantly predictive scores based on clinical factors in the prediction of subsequent thyroid cancers in childhood cancer survivors of European ancestry [119]. Future studies should investigate the combined effect of PRS and exposure to lifestyle and environmental factors in order to enhance individualized DTC risk prediction. There is also a need to extend the DTC PRS to other ethnic groups.

4. Conclusion

Despite the solid evidence for heritability of thyroid cancer, only a handful of variants have been significantly associated with an increased risk of DTC representing the most common form of thyroid cancer. The high heritability of the disease is likely due to the contribution of rare high-penetrance variants in some cases and the combination of common low-penetrance variants in others, as well as the influence of common shared environmental factors in DTC-prone families or in specific groups of the general population. So far, efforts to identify DTC predisposing genes outside of syndromic FNMTC led to the identification of mainly low-to-moderate penetrance genes, and routine genetic testing for these genes is not recommended. Further large studies to characterize their penetrance and function and to identify new DTC-associated loci or alternative hereditary mechanisms such as epigenetic modifications are required to improve our understanding of DTC tumorigenesis. Ultimately, risk prediction models integrating family history of DTC, PRS, and some modifiable risk factors (obesity, exposure to ionizing radiations from medical diagnostic procedure, etc.) may help stratify individuals according to their risk of developing DTC, which can be useful for elaborating screening policies. Moreover, inherited genetic factors can also impact the final outcome of the disease such as histological subtypes, localization of metastases, or molecular profiling of the tumor, and their characterization can help to predict effectiveness of the initial treatment [120].

Author details

Fabienne Lesueur[1] and Thérèse Truong[2]*

1 Inserm, U900, Institut Curie, PSL University, Mines ParisTech, Paris, France

2 University Paris-Saclay, UVSQ, Inserm, Gustave Roussy, CESP, Team “Exposome and Heredity”, Villejuif, France

*Address all correspondence to: therese.truong@inserm.fr

References

[1] Chrisoulidou A, Boudina M, Tzemailas A, Doumala E, Iliadou PK, Patakiouta F, et al. Histological subtype is the most important determinant of survival in metastatic papillary thyroid cancer. Thyroid Research. 2011;**4**(1):12. DOI: 10.1186/1756-6614-4-12

[2] Jemal A, Siegel R, Xu J, Ward E. Cancer statistics, 2010. CA: A Cancer Journal for Clinicians. 2010;**60**(5):277-300. DOI: 10.3322/caac.20073

[3] Bray F, Ferlay J, Soerjomataram I, Siegel R, Torre L, Jemal A. Global cancer statistics 2018: GLOBOCAN estimates of incidence and mortality worldwide for 36 cancers in 185 countries. CA: A Cancer Journal for Clinicians. 2018;**68**(6):394-424

[4] Truong T, Rougier Y, Dubourdieu D, Guihenneuc-Jouyaux C, Orsi L, Hémon D, et al. Time trends and geographic variations for thyroid cancer in New Caledonia, a very high incidence area (1985-1999). European Journal of Cancer Prevention. 2007;**16**(1995):62-70

[5] Ito Y, Nikiforov YE, Schlumberger M, Vigneri R. Increasing incidence of thyroid cancer: Controversies explored. Nature Reviews. Endocrinology. 2013;**9**(3):178-184. DOI: 10.1038/nrendo.2012.257

[6] Goldgar DE, Easton DF, Cannon-Albright LA, Skolnick MH. Systematic population-based assessment of cancer risk in first-degree relatives of cancer probands. Journal of the National Cancer Institute. 1994;**86**(21):1600-1608

[7] Dong C, Hemminki K. Modification of cancer risks in offspring by sibling and parental cancers from 2,112,616 nuclear families. International Journal of Cancer. 2001;**92**(1):144-150

[8] Hemminki K, Dong C. Familial relationships in thyroid cancer by histo-pathological type. International Journal of Cancer. 2000;**85**(2):201-205

[9] Hrafnkelsson J, Tulinius H, Jonasson JG, Sigvaldason H. Familial non-medullary thyroid cancer in Iceland. Journal of Medical Genetics. 2001;**38**(3):189-191. DOI: 10.1136/jmg.38.3.189

[10] Frich L, Glattre E, Akslen LA. Familial occurrence of nonmedullary thyroid cancer: A population-based study of 5673 first-degree relatives of thyroid cancer patients from Norway. Cancer Epidemiology, Biomarkers & Prevention. 2001;**10**(2):113-117

[11] Lin HT, Liu FC, Lin SF, Kuo CF, Chen YY, Yu HP. Familial aggregation and heritability of nonmedullary thyroid cancer in an asian population: A nationwide cohort study. The Journal of Clinical Endocrinology and Metabolism. 2020;**105**(7). DOI: 10.1210/clinem/dgaa191

[12] Xing M. Molecular pathogenesis and mechanisms of thyroid cancer. Nature Reviews. Cancer. 2013;**13**(3):184-199. DOI: 10.1038/nrc3431

[13] Romei C, Ciampi R, Elisei R. A comprehensive overview of the role of the RET proto-oncogene in thyroid carcinoma. Nature Reviews. Endocrinology. 2016;**12**(4):192-202. DOI: 10.1038/nrendo.2016.11

[14] Hedayati M, Zarif Yeganeh M, Sheikholeslami S, Afsari F. Diversity of mutations in the RET proto-oncogene

and its oncogenic mechanism in medullary thyroid cancer. Critical Reviews in Clinical Laboratory Sciences. 2016;**53**(4):217-227. DOI: 10.3109/10408363.2015.1129529

[15] Accardo G, Conzo G, Esposito D, Gambardella C, Mazzella M, Castaldo F, et al. Genetics of medullary thyroid cancer: An overview. International Journal of Surgery. 2017;**41**(Suppl. 1):S2-S6. DOI: 10.1016/j.ijsu.2017.02.064

[16] Hincza K, Kowalik A, Kowalska A. Current knowledge of germline genetic risk factors for the development of non-medullary thyroid cancer. Genes (Basel). 2019;**10**(7):482. DOI: 10.3390/genes10070482

[17] Schultz KAP, Rednam SP, Kamihara J, Doros L, Achatz MI, Wasserman JD, et al. PTEN, DICER1, FH, and their associated tumor susceptibility syndromes: Clinical features, genetics, and surveillance recommendations in childhood. Clinical Cancer Research. 2017;**23**(12):e76-e82. DOI: 10.1158/1078-0432.CCR-17-0629

[18] Son EJ, Nose V. Familial follicular cell-derived thyroid carcinoma. Frontiers in Endocrinology. 2012;**3**:61. DOI: 10.3389/fendo.2012.00061

[19] Legrand MA, Raverot G, Nicolino M, Chapurlat R. GNAS mutated thyroid carcinoma in a patient with Mc Cune Albright syndrome. Bone Reports. 2020;**13**:100299. DOI: 10.1016/j.bonr.2020.100299

[20] Lacka K, Maciejewski A, Stawny B, Lacki JK. Follicular thyroid cancer in a patient with pendred syndrome. Annales d'Endocrinologie. 2021;**82**(6):622-624. DOI: 10.1016/j.ando.2021.05.001

[21] Malchoff CD, Malchoff DM. Familial nonmedullary thyroid carcinoma. Cancer Control. 2006;**13**(2):106-110

[22] Malchoff CD, Sarfarazi M, Tendler B, Forouhar F, Whalen G, Joshi V, et al. Papillary thyroid carcinoma associated with papillary renal neoplasia: Genetic linkage analysis of a distinct heritable tumor syndrome. The Journal of Clinical Endocrinology and Metabolism. 2000;**85**(5):1758-1764

[23] Rio Frio T, Bahubeshi A, Kanellopoulou C, Hamel N, Niedziela M, Sabbaghian N, et al. DICER1 mutations in familial multinodular goiter with and without ovarian Sertoli-Leydig cell tumors. JAMA. 2011;**305**(1):68-77. DOI: 10.1001/jama.2010.1910

[24] Moses W, Weng J, Kebebew E. Prevalence, clinicopathologic features, and somatic genetic mutation profile in familial versus sporadic nonmedullary thyroid cancer. Thyroid. 2011;**21**(4):367-371. DOI: 10.1089/thy.2010.0256

[25] Pitoia F, Cross G, Salvai ME, Abelleira E, Niepomniszcze H. Patients with familial non-medullary thyroid cancer have an outcome similar to that of patients with sporadic papillary thyroid tumors. Arquivos Brasileiros de Endocrinologia & Metabologia. 2011;**55**(3):219-223. DOI: 10.1590/s0004-27302011000300007

[26] Capezzone M, Fralassi N, Secchi C, Cantara S, Brilli L, Pilli T, et al. Long-term clinical outcome in familial and sporadic papillary thyroid carcinoma. The European Thyroid Journal. 2020;**9**(4):213-220. DOI: 10.1159/000506955

[27] Park YJ, Ahn HY, Choi HS, Kim KW, Park DJ, Cho BY. The long-term outcomes of the second generation of familial nonmedullary thyroid carcinoma are more aggressive than sporadic cases. Thyroid. 2012;**22**(4):356-362. DOI: 10.1089/thy.2011.0163

[28] Dinarvand P, Davaro EP, Doan JV, Ising ME, Evans NR, Phillips NJ, et al.

Familial adenomatous polyposis syndrome: An update and review of extraintestinal manifestations. Archives of Pathology & Laboratory Medicine. 2019;**143**(11):1382-1398. DOI: 10.5858/arpa.2018-0570-RA

[29] Harach HR, Williams GT, Williams ED. Familial adenomatous polyposis associated thyroid carcinoma: A distinct type of follicular cell neoplasm. Histopathology. 1994;**25**(6):549-561. DOI: 10.1111/j.1365-2559.1994.tb01374.x

[30] Soravia C, Sugg SL, Berk T, Mitri A, Cheng H, Gallinger S, et al. Familial adenomatous polyposis-associated thyroid cancer: A clinical, pathological, and molecular genetics study. The American Journal of Pathology. 1999;**154**(1):127-135. DOI: 10.1016/S0002-9440(10)65259-5

[31] Cameselle-Teijeiro J, Chan JK. Cribriform-morular variant of papillary carcinoma: A distinctive variant representing the sporadic counterpart of familial adenomatous polyposis-associated thyroid carcinoma? Modern Pathology. 1999;**12**(4):400-411

[32] Herraiz M, Barbesino G, Faquin W, Chan-Smutko G, Patel D, Shannon KM, et al. Prevalence of thyroid cancer in familial adenomatous polyposis syndrome and the role of screening ultrasound examinations. Clinical Gastroenterology and Hepatology. 2007;**5**(3):367-373. DOI: 10.1016/j.cgh.2006.10.019

[33] Crippa S, Saletti P, Barizzi J, Mazzucchelli L. The clinical management in familial adenomatous polyposis deserves continuous monitoring for thyroid carcinoma. BML Case Reports. 2012;**2012**:1-3. DOI: 10.1136/bcr-2012-007046

[34] Tan MH, Mester JL, Ngeow J, Rybicki LA, Orloff MS, Eng C. Lifetime cancer risks in individuals with germline PTEN mutations. Clinical Cancer Research. 2012;**18**(2):400-407. DOI: 10.1158/1078-0432.CCR-11-2283

[35] Ngeow J, Mester J, Rybicki LA, Ni Y, Milas M, Eng C. Incidence and clinical characteristics of thyroid cancer in prospective series of individuals with Cowden and Cowden-like syndrome characterized by germline PTEN, SDH, or KLLN alterations. The Journal of Clinical Endocrinology and Metabolism. 2011;**96**(12):E2063-E2071. DOI: 10.1210/jc.2011-1616

[36] Bertherat J, Horvath A, Groussin L, Grabar S, Boikos S, Cazabat L, et al. Mutations in regulatory subunit type 1A of cyclic adenosine 5'-monophosphate-dependent protein kinase (PRKAR1A): Phenotype analysis in 353 patients and 80 different genotypes. The Journal of Clinical Endocrinology and Metabolism. 2009;**94**(6):2085-2091. DOI: 10.1210/jc.2008-2333

[37] Bossis I, Stratakis CA. Minireview: PRKAR1A: Normal and abnormal functions. Endocrinology. 2004;**145**(12):5452-5458. DOI: 10.1210/en.2004-0900

[38] Nikiforov YE. RET/PTC rearrangement in thyroid tumors. Endocrine Pathology. 2002;**13**(1):3-16. DOI: 10.1385/ep:13:1:03

[39] Yu CE, Oshima J, Hisama FM, Matthews S, Trask BJ, Schellenberg GD. A YAC, P1, and cosmid contig and 17 new polymorphic markers for the Werner syndrome region at 8p12-p21. Genomics. 1996;**35**(3):431-440. DOI: 10.1006/geno.1996.0382

[40] Lauper JM, Krause A, Vaughan TL, Monnat RJ Jr. Spectrum and risk of neoplasia in Werner syndrome: A systematic review. PLoS One.

2013;**8**(4):e59709. DOI: 10.1371/journal.pone.0059709

[41] Slade I, Bacchelli C, Davies H, Murray A, Abbaszadeh F, Hanks S, et al. DICER1 syndrome: Clarifying the diagnosis, clinical features and management implications of a pleiotropic tumour predisposition syndrome. Journal of Medical Genetics. 2011;**48**(4):273-278. DOI: 10.1136/jmg.2010.083790

[42] Fuziwara CS, Kimura ET. MicroRNAs in thyroid development, function and tumorigenesis. Molecular and Cellular Endocrinology. 2017;**456**:44-50. DOI: 10.1016/j.mce.2016.12.017

[43] Khan NE, Bauer AJ, KAP S, Doros L, Decastro RM, Ling A, et al. Quantification of thyroid cancer and multinodular goiter risk in the DICER1 syndrome: A family-based cohort study. The Journal of Clinical Endocrinology and Metabolism. 2017;**102**(5):1614-1622. DOI: 10.1210/jc.2016-2954

[44] Bignell GR, Canzian F, Shayeghi M, Stark M, Shugart YY, Biggs P, et al. Familial nontoxic multinodular thyroid goiter locus maps to chromosome 14q but does not account for familial nonmedullary thyroid cancer. American Journal of Human Genetics. 1997;**61**(5):1123-1130

[45] Lesueur F, Stark M, Tocco T, Ayadi H, Delisle MJ, Goldgar DE, et al. Genetic heterogeneity in familial nonmedullary thyroid carcinoma: Exclusion of linkage to RET, MNG1, and TCO in 56 families. NMTC consortium. The Journal of Clinical Endocrinology and Metabolism. 1999;**84**(6):2157-2162

[46] Diquigiovanni C, Bergamini C, Evangelisti C, Isidori F, Vettori A, Tiso N, et al. Mutant MYO1F alters the mitochondrial network and induces tumor proliferation in thyroid cancer. International Journal of Cancer. 2018;**143**(7):1706-1719. DOI: 10.1002/ijc.31548

[47] Canzian F, Amati P, Harach HR, Kraimps JL, Lesueur F, Barbier J, et al. A gene predisposing to familial thyroid tumors with cell oxyphilia maps to chromosome 19p13.2. American Journal of Human Genetics. 1998;**63**(6):1743-1748

[48] McKay JD, Lesueur F, Jonard L, Pastore A, Williamson J, Hoffman L, et al. Localization of a susceptibility gene for familial nonmedullary thyroid carcinoma to chromosome 2q21. American Journal of Human Genetics. 2001;**69**(2):440-446

[49] Cavaco BM, Batista PF, Sobrinho LG, Leite V. Mapping a new familial thyroid epithelial neoplasia susceptibility locus to chromosome 8p23.1-p22 by high-density single-nucleotide polymorphism genome-wide linkage analysis. The Journal of Clinical Endocrinology and Metabolism. 2008;**93**(11):4426-4430

[50] He H, Nagy R, Liyanarachchi S, Jiao H, Li W, Suster S, et al. A susceptibility locus for papillary thyroid carcinoma on chromosome 8q24. Cancer Research. 2009;**69**(2):625-631

[51] He H, Bronisz A, Liyanarachchi S, Nagy R, Li W, Huang Y, et al. SRGAP1 is a candidate gene for papillary thyroid carcinoma susceptibility. The Journal of Clinical Endocrinology and Metabolism. 2013;**98**(5):E973-E980. DOI: 10.1210/jc.2012-3823

[52] He H, Li W, Wu D, Nagy R, Liyanarachchi S, Akagi K, et al. Ultra-rare mutation in long-range enhancer predisposes to thyroid carcinoma with high penetrance. PLoS One. 2013;**8**(5):e61920. DOI: 10.1371/journal.pone.0061920

[53] Gara SK, Jia L, Merino MJ, Agarwal SK, Zhang L, Cam M, et al. Germline HABP2 mutation causing familial nonmedullary thyroid cancer. The New England Journal of Medicine. 2015;**373**(5):448-455. DOI: 10.1056/NEJMoa1502449

[54] Tomsic J, He H, de la Chapelle A. HABP2 mutation and nonmedullary thyroid cancer. The New England Journal of Medicine. 2015;**373**(21):2086. DOI: 10.1056/NEJMc1511631

[55] Tomsic J, He H, Akagi K, Liyanarachchi S, Pan Q, Bertani B, et al. A germline mutation in SRRM2, a splicing factor gene, is implicated in papillary thyroid carcinoma predisposition. Scientific Reports. 2015;**5**:10566. DOI: 10.1038/srep10566

[56] Ye F, Gao H, Xiao L, Zuo Z, Liu Y, Zhao Q, et al. Whole exome and target sequencing identifies MAP2K5 as novel susceptibility gene for familial non-medullary thyroid carcinoma. International Journal of Cancer. 2019;**144**(6):1321-1330. DOI: 10.1002/ijc.31825

[57] Cirello V, Colombo C, Persani L, Fugazzola L. Absence of the MAP2K5 germline variants c.G961A and c.T1100C in a wide series of familial nonmedullary thyroid carcinoma Italian families. International Journal of Cancer. 2019;**145**(2):600. DOI: 10.1002/ijc.32244

[58] Orois A, Gara SK, Mora M, Halperin I, Martinez S, Alfayate R, et al. NOP53 as a candidate modifier locus for familial non-medullary thyroid cancer. Genes (Basel). 2019;**10**(11). DOI: 10.3390/genes10110899

[59] Srivastava A, Kumar A, Giangiobbe S, Bonora E, Hemminki K, Forsti A, et al. Whole genome sequencing of familial non-medullary thyroid cancer identifies germline alterations in MAPK/ERK and PI3K/AKT signaling pathways. Biomolecules. 2019;**9**(10). DOI: 10.3390/biom9100605

[60] He H, Li W, Comiskey DF, Liyanarachchi S, Nieminen TT, Wang Y, et al. A truncating germline mutation of TINF2 in individuals with thyroid cancer or melanoma results in longer telomeres. Thyroid. 2020;**30**(2):204-213. DOI: 10.1089/thy.2019.0156

[61] Wang Y, Liyanarachchi S, Miller KE, Nieminen TT, Comiskey DF Jr, Li W, et al. Identification of rare variants predisposing to thyroid cancer. Thyroid. 2019;**29**(7):946-955. DOI: 10.1089/thy.2018.0736

[62] Wilson TL, Hattangady N, Lerario AM, Williams C, Koeppe E, Quinonez S, et al. A new POT1 germline mutation-expanding the spectrum of POT1-associated cancers. Familial Cancer. 2017;**16**(4):561-566. DOI: 10.1007/s10689-017-9984-y

[63] Orois A, Badenas C, Reverter JL, Lopez V, Potrony M, Mora M, et al. Lack of mutations in POT1 gene in selected families with familial non-medullary thyroid cancer. Hormone Therapy for Cancer. 2020;**11**(2):111-116. DOI: 10.1007/s12672-020-00383-5

[64] Srivastava A, Miao B, Skopelitou D, Kumar V, Kumar A, Paramasivam N, et al. A germline mutation in the POT1 gene is a candidate for familial non-medullary thyroid cancer. Cancers (Basel). 2020;**12**(6):1441. DOI: 10.3390/cancers12061441

[65] Adjadj E, Schlumberger M, Vathaire F De. Germ-line DNA polymorphisms and susceptibility to differentiated thyroid cancer. The Lancet Oncology 2009;10(2):181-190. DOI: 10.1016/S1470-2045(09)70020-8

[66] Landa I, Robledo M. Association studies in thyroid cancer susceptibility:

Are we on the right track? Journal of Molecular Endocrinology. 2011;**47**:R43-R58. DOI: 10.1530/JME-11-0005

[67] Figlioli G, Elisei R, Romei C, Melaiu O, Cipollini M, Bambi F, et al. A comprehensive meta-analysis of case – control association studies to evaluate polymorphisms associated with the risk of differentiated thyroid carcinoma. Cancer Causes & Control. 2016;**25**(4):700-713. DOI: 10.1158/1055-9965.EPI-15-0652

[68] Gudmundsson J, Sulem P, Gudbjartsson DF, Jonasson JG, Sigurdsson A, Bergthorsson JT, et al. Common variants on 9q22.33 and 14q13.3 predispose to thyroid cancer in European populations. Nature Genetics. 2009;**41**(4):460-464. DOI: 10.1038/ng.339

[69] Takahashi M, Saenko VA, Rogounovitch TI, Kawaguchi T, Drozd VM, Takigawa-Imamura H, et al. The FOXE1 locus is a major genetic determinant for radiation-related thyroid carcinoma in Chernobyl. Human Molecular Genetics. 2010;**19**(12):2516-2523. DOI: 10.1093/hmg/ddq123

[70] Köhler A, Chen B, Gemignani F, Elisei R, Romei C, Figlioli G, et al. Genome-wide association study on differentiated thyroid cancer. The Journal of Clinical Endocrinology and Metabolism. 2013;**98**(10):E1674-E1681. DOI: 10.1210/jc.2013-1941

[71] Mancikova V, Cruz R, Inglada-Pérez L, Fernández-Rozadilla C, Landa I, Cameselle-Teijeiro J, et al. Thyroid cancer GWAS identifies 10q26.12 and 6q14.1 as novel susceptibility loci and reveals genetic heterogeneity among populations. International Journal of Cancer. 2015;**137**(8):1870-1878. DOI: 10.1002/ijc.29557

[72] Gudmundsson J, Thorleifsson G, Sigurdsson JK, Stefansdottir L, Jonasson JG, Gudjonsson SA, et al. A genome-wide association study yields five novel thyroid cancer risk loci. Nature Communications. 2017;**8**:14517. DOI: 10.1038/ncomms14517

[73] Truong T, Lesueur F, Sugier P, Guibon J, Xhaard C, Karimi M, et al. Multiethnic genome-wide association study of differentiated thyroid cancer in the EPITHYR consortium. International Journal of Cancer. 2021;**148**(12):2935-2946. DOI: 10.1002/ijc.33488

[74] Son HY, Hwangbo Y, Yoo SK, Im SW, Yang SD, Kwak SJ, et al. Genome-wide association and expression quantitative trait loci studies identify multiple susceptibility loci for thyroid cancer. Nature Communications. 2017;**8**:15966. DOI: 10.1038/ncomms15966

[75] Jones AM, Howarth KM, Martin L, Gorman M, Mihai R, Moss L, et al. Thyroid cancer susceptibility polymorphisms: Confirmation of loci on chromosomes 9q22 and 14q13, validation of a recessive 8q24 locus and failure to replicate a locus on 5q24. Journal of Medical Genetics. 2012;**49, 63**(3):158. DOI: 10.1136/jmedgenet-2011-100586

[76] Tomaz RA, Sousa I, Silva JG, Santos C, Teixeira MR, Leite V, et al. FOXE1 polymorphisms are associated with familial and sporadic nonmedullary thyroid cancer susceptibility. Clinical Endocrinology (Oxf). 2012;77(6):926-933. DOI: 10.1111/j.1365-2265.2012.04505.x

[77] Penna-Martinez M, Epp F, Kahles H, Ramos-Lopez E, Hinsch N, Hansmann ML, et al. FOXE1 association with differentiated thyroid cancer and its progression. Thyroid. 2014;**24**(5):845-851

[78] Jendrzejewski J, Liyanarachchi S, Nagy R, Senter L, Wakely PE, Thomas A, et al. Papillary thyroid

carcinoma: Association between germline DNA variant markers and clinical parameters. Thyroid. 2016;**26**(9):1276-1284

[79] Tcheandjieu C, Lesueur F, Sanchez M, Baron-Dubourdieu D, Guizard AV, Mulot C, et al. Fine-mapping of two differentiated thyroid carcinoma susceptibility loci at 9q22.33 and 14q13.3 detects novel candidate functional SNPs in Europeans from metropolitan France and Melanesians from New Caledonia. International Journal of Cancer. 2016;**139**(3):617-627

[80] Kula D, Kalemba M, Puch Z, Polaska J, Swierniak M, Rusinek D, et al. Age at diagnosis and gender modify the risk of 9q22 and 14q13 polymorphisms for papillary thyroid carcinoma. Endokrynologia Polska. 2017;**68**(3): 283-289

[81] Nikitski AV, Rogounovitch TI, Bychkov A, Takahashi M, Yoshiura KI, Mitsutake N, et al. Genotype analyses in the Japanese and belarusian populations reveal independent effects of rs965513 and rs1867277 but do not support the role of FOXE1 polyalanine tract length in conferring risk for papillary thyroid carcinoma. Thyroid. 2017;**27**(2):224-235

[82] Gudmundsson J, Sulem P, Gudbjartsson DF, Jonasson JG, Masson G, He H, et al. Discovery of common variants associated with low TSH levels and thyroid cancer risk. Nature Genetics. 2012;**44**(3):319-322

[83] Matsuse M, Takahashi M, Mitsutake N, Nishihara E, Hirokawa M, Kawaguchi T, et al. The FOXE1 and NKX2-1 loci are associated with susceptibility to papillary thyroid carcinoma in the Japanese population. Journal of Medical Genetics. 2011;**48**(9):645-648. DOI: 10.1136/jmedgenet-2011-100063

[84] Wang YL, Feng SH, Guo SC, Wei WJ, Li DS, Wang Y, et al. Confirmation of papillary thyroid cancer susceptibility loci identified by genome-wide association studies of chromosomes 14q13, 9q22, 2q35 and 8p12 in a Chinese population. Journal of Medical Genetics. 2013;**50**(10):689-695. DOI: 10.1136/jmedgenet-2013-101687

[85] Guo S, Wang YL, Li Y, Jin L, Xiong M, Ji QH, et al. Significant SNPs have limited prediction ability for thyroid cancer. Cancer Medicine. 2014;**3**(3):731-735. DOI: 10.1002/cam4.211

[86] Maillard S, Damiola F, Clero E, Pertesi M, Robinot N, Rachédi F, et al. Common variants at 9q22.33, 14q13.3, and ATM loci, and risk of differentiated thyroid cancer in the French Polynesian population. PLoS One. 2015;**10**(4):e0123700. DOI: 10.1371/JOURNAL.PONE.0123700

[87] Pereda CM, Lesueur F, Pertesi M, Robinot N, Lence-Anta JJ, Turcios S, et al. Common variants at the 9q22.33, 14q13.3 and ATM loci, and risk of differentiated thyroid cancer in the Cuban population. BMC Genetics. 2015;**16**:22. DOI: 10.1186/s12863-015-0180-5

[88] Estrada-Florez AP, Bohórquez ME, Sahasrabudhe R, Prieto R, Lott P, Duque CS, et al. Clinical features of Hispanic thyroid cancer cases and the role of known genetic variants on disease risk. Medicine (Baltimore). 2016;**95**(32):e4148. DOI: 10.1097/MD.0000000000004148

[89] Mussazhanova Z, Rogounovitch TI, Saenko VA, Krykpayeva A, Espenbetova M, Azizov B, et al. The contribution of genetic variants to the risk of papillary thyroid carcinoma in the kazakh population: Study of common single nucleotide polymorphisms and their clinicopathological correlations.

Frontiers in Endocrinology (Lausanne). 2020;**11**:543500. DOI: 10.3389/fendo.2020.543500

[90] Landa I, Ruiz-Llorente S, Montero-Conde C, Inglada-Perez L, Schiavi F, Leskela S, et al. The variant rs1867277 in FOXE1 gene confers thyroid cancer susceptibility through the recruitment of USF1/USF2 transcription factors. PLoS Genetics. 2009;**5**(9):e1000637

[91] He H, Li W, Liyanarachchi S, Jendrzejewski J, Srinivas M, Davuluri RV, et al. Genetic predisposition to papillary thyroid carcinoma: Involvement of FOXE1, TSHR, and a novel lincRNA Gene, PTCSC2. The Journal of Clinical Endocrinology and Metabolism. 2015;**100**(1):E164-E172

[92] Wei WJ, Lu ZW, Wang Y, Zhu YX, Wang YL, Ji QH. Clinical significance of papillary thyroid cancer risk loci identified by genome-wide association studies. Cancer Genetics. 2015;**208**(3):68-75

[93] Jendrzejewski J, Liyanarachchi S, Eiterman A, Thomas A, He H, Nagy R, et al. Fine mapping of 14q13 reveals novel variants associated with different histological subtypes of papillary thyroid carcinoma. International Journal of Cancer. 2019;**144**(3):503-512. DOI: 10.1002/ijc.31933

[94] Rogounovitch TI, Bychkov A, Takahashi M, Mitsutake N, Nakashima M, Nikitski AV, et al. The common genetic variant rs944289 on chromosome 14q13.3 associates with risk of both malignant and benign thyroid tumors in the Japanese population. Thyroid. 2015;**25**(3):333-340

[95] Jendrzejewski J, He H, Radomska HS, Li W, Tomsic J, Liyanarachchi S, et al. The polymorphism rs944289 predisposes to papillary thyroid carcinoma through a large intergenic noncoding RNA gene of tumor suppressor type. Proceedings of the National Academy of Sciences of the United States of America. 2012;**109**(22):8646-8651. DOI: 10.1073/PNAS.1205654109

[96] Guibon J, Sugier PE, Kulkarni O, Karimi M, Bacq-Daian D, Besse C, et al. Fine–mapping of two differentiated thyroid carcinoma susceptibility loci at 2q35 and 8p12 in Europeans, Melanesians and Polynesians. Oncotarget. 2021;**12**(5):493-506. DOI: 10.18632/ONCOTARGET.27888

[97] Michailidou K, Beesley J, Lindstrom S, Canisius S, Dennis J, Lush MJ, et al. Genome-wide association analysis of more than 120,000 individuals identifies 15 new susceptibility loci for breast cancer. Nature Genetics. 2015;**47**(4):373-380. DOI: 10.1038/ng.3242

[98] Liyanarachchi S, Wojcicka A, Li W, Czetwertynska M, Stachlewska E, Nagy R, et al. Cumulative risk impact of five genetic variants associated with papillary thyroid carcinoma. Thyroid. 2013;**23**(12):1532-1540. DOI: 10.1089/thy.2013.0102

[99] He H, Li W, Liyanarachchi S, Wang Y, Yu L, Genutis LK, et al. The role of NRG1 in the predisposition to papillary thyroid carcinoma. The Journal of Clinical Endocrinology and Metabolism. 2018;**103**(4):1369-1379. DOI: 10.1210/JC.2017-01798

[100] Pooley KA, Bojesen SE, Weischer M, Nielsen SF, Thompson D, Amin Al Olama A, et al. A genome-wide association scan (GWAS) for mean telomere length within the COGS project: Identified loci show little association with hormone-related cancer risk. Human Molecular Genetics.

2013;**22**(24):5056-5064. DOI: 10.1093/HMG/DDT355

[101] Li Y, Xiang C, Shen N, Deng L, Luo X, Yuan P, et al. Functional polymorphisms on chromosome 5p15.33 disturb telomere biology and confer the risk of non-small cell lung cancer in Chinese population. Molecular Carcinogenesis. 2019;**58**(6):913-921. DOI: 10.1002/MC.22980

[102] Rode L, Nordestgaard BG, Bojesen SE. Long telomeres and cancer risk among 95 568 individuals from the general population. International Journal of Epidemiology. 2016;**45**(5):1634-1643. DOI: 10.1093/IJE/DYW179

[103] Terry KL, Tworoger SS, Vitonis AF, Wong J, Titus-Ernstoff L, De Vivo I, et al. Telomere length and genetic variation in telomere maintenance genes in relation to ovarian cancer risk. Cancer Epidemiology, Biomarkers & Prevention. 2012;**21**(3):504-512

[104] Phelan CM, Kuchenbaecker KB, Tyrer JP, Kar SP, Lawrenson K, Winham SJ, et al. Identification of 12 new susceptibility loci for different histotypes of epithelial ovarian cancer. Nature Genetics. 2017;**49**(5):680-691. DOI: 10.1038/NG.3826

[105] Turner AW, Martinuk A, Silva A, Lau P, Nikpay M, Eriksson P, et al. Functional analysis of a novel genome-wide association study signal in SMAD3 that confers protection from coronary artery disease. Arteriosclerosis, Thrombosis, and Vascular Biology. 2016;**36**(5):972-983. DOI: 10.1161/ATVBAHA.116.307294

[106] Wu M, Assassi S, Salazar GA, Pedroza C, Gorlova OY, Chen WV, et al. Genetic susceptibility loci of idiopathic interstitial pneumonia do not represent risk for systemic sclerosis: A case control study in Caucasian patients. Arthritis Research & Therapy. 2016;**18**(1). DOI: 10.1186/S13075-016-0923-3

[107] Rosenthal EA, Crosslin DR, Gordon AS, Carrell DS, Stanaway IB, Larson EB, et al. Association between triglycerides, known risk SNVs and conserved rare variation in SLC25A40 in a multi-ancestry cohort. BMC Medical Genomics. 2021;**14**(1). DOI: 10.1186/S12920-020-00854-2

[108] Song SS, Huang S, Park S. Association of polygenetic risk scores related to cell differentiation and inflammation with thyroid cancer risk and genetic interaction with dietary intake. Cancers (Basel). 2021;**13**(7):1510. DOI: 10.3390/cancers13071510

[109] Hao R, Han P, Zhang L, Bi Y, Yan J, Li H, et al. Genetic polymorphisms in the PCNXL2 gene are risk factors for thyroid cancer in the Chinese population. Future Oncology. 2021;**17**(34):4677-4686. DOI: 10.2217/FON-2021-0748

[110] Ren W, Xu C, Wang S, Li H, Dai H, Yang F, et al. The effect of VAV3 polymorphisms on thyroid cancer. Endocrine. 2022;**75**(1):178-184. DOI: 10.1007/s12020-021-02827-6

[111] Liu Y, Shi F. Associations of telomerase reverse transcriptase rs10069690 and rs2736100 polymorphisms with papillary thyroid carcinoma. European Journal of Cancer Prevention. 2020:259-265. DOI: 10.1097/CEJ.0000000000000536

[112] He G, Song T, Zhang Y, Chen X, Xiong W, Chen H, et al. TERT rs10069690 polymorphism and cancers risk: A meta-analysis. Molecular Genetics & Genomic Medicine. 2019;**7**(10):e00903. DOI: 10.1002/MGG3.903

[113] dos Santos ICC, Genre J, Marques D, da Silva AMG, dos Santos JC, de Araújo JNG, et al. A new panel of SNPs to assess thyroid carcinoma risk: A pilot study in a Brazilian admixture population. BMC Medical Genetics. 2017;**18**(1):140. DOI: 10.1186/S12881-017-0502-8

[114] Figlioli G, Chen B, Elisei R, Romei C, Campo C, Cipollini M, et al. Novel genetic variants in differentiated thyroid cancer and assessment of the cumulative risk. Scientific Reports. 2015;**5**:8922

[115] Graff RE, Cavazos TB, Thai KK, Kachuri L, Rashkin SR, Hoffman JD, et al. Cross-cancer evaluation of polygenic risk scores for 16 cancer types in two large cohorts. Nature Communications. 2021;**12**(1). DOI: 10.1038/s41467-021-21288-z

[116] Park J, Choi J yeob, Choi J, Chung S, Song N, Park SK, et al. Gene-environment interactions relevant to estrogen and risk of breast cancer: Can gene-environment interactions be detected only among candidate SNPs from genome-wide association studies? Cancers (Basel). 2021;**13**(10):2370

[117] Wang L, Desai H, Verma SS, Le A, Hausler R, Verma A, et al. Performance of polygenic risk scores for cancer prediction in a racially diverse academic biobank. Genetics in Medicine. 2022;**24**(3):601-609. DOI: 10.1016/j.gim.2021.10.015

[118] Liyanarachchi S, Gudmundsson J, Ferkingstad E, He H, Jonasson JG, Tragante V, et al. Assessing thyroid cancer risk using polygenic risk scores. Proceedings of the National Academy of Sciences of the United States of America. 2020;**117**(11):5997-6002. DOI: 10.1073/pnas.1919976117

[119] Song N, Liu Q, Wilson CL, Sapkota Y, Ehrhardt MJ, Gibson TM, et al. Polygenic risk score improves risk stratification and prediction of subsequent thyroid cancer after childhood cancer. Cancer Epidemiology, Biomarkers & Prevention. 2021;**30**(11):2096-2104. DOI: 10.1158/1055-9965.EPI-21-0448

[120] Jendrzejewski JP, Sworczak K, Comiskey DF, de la Chapelle A. Clinical implications of GWAS variants associated with differentiated thyroid cancer. Endokrynologia Polska. 2019;**70**(5):423-429. DOI: 10.5603/EP.a2019.0027

Chapter 2

RET Proto-Oncogene Mutations: Impact on Diagnosis, Treatment and Prognosis of MTC

Shabnam Heydarzadeh and Mehdi Hedayati

Abstract

Variants of MTC result from different mutations in exons of the RET gene. RET proto-oncogene is activated by a DNA rearrangement and it is one of the first tyrosine kinase receptor (RTK) proteins found to play a role in neoplasia. Early detection using genetic screening has become the gold standard of therapy, followed by prophylactic thyroidectomy. RET-kinase inhibitors have been developed recently for the treatment of MTC and are currently at various phases of pre- and clinical trials. Numerous autosomal dominantly inherited mutations have been demonstrated to activate RET constitutively. These mutations in separate populations are believed to be correlated with a rather heterogeneous prototype across countries. As such, one objective of this study was to demonstrate a geographical pattern of RET mutations in various populations. Advances in RET genetic screening have facilitated for the rapid recognition of hereditary MTCs and prophylactic thyroidectomy for relatives who may not show signs of the disease. In this chapter, we will discuss oncogenic RET signaling, RET inhibitors and the major RET mutations found in MTC and the necessity of RET genetic screening for the early diagnosis of MTC patients, using American Thyroid Association guidelines and genotype-phenotype correlation.

Keywords: medullary thyroid cancer, RET proto-oncogene, RET mutation, RET signaling, RET inhibitors

1. Introduction

The medullary thyroid carcinoma (MTC) is one of the most aggressive kinds of thyroid cancer. It is a neuroendocrine tumor and is notably distinct from differentiated thyroid carcinoma. MTC accounts for 5–10% of all thyroid malignancies and occurs in both sporadic (75%) and inherited (25% of cases) forms [1, 2]. The latter exhibits an autosomal dominant inheritance pattern with varying expressivity and age-dependent penetrance [3, 4]. RET (REarranged during Transfection) proto-oncogene is essential for the molecular pathogenesis of hereditary MTCs [5].

The human RET proto-oncogene encodes a transmembrane receptor tyrosine kinase that transmits growth and differentiation signals. Extracellular binding of ligands and coreceptors, receptor dimerization via the cysteine-rich domain, and intracellular autophosphorylation of the tyrosine kinase catalytic domain are required for RET function. RET can be activated oncogenically *in vivo* and *in vitro* by cytogenetic rearrangement. RET gene mutations have been identified in a variety of human disorders, including PTC (Papillary thyroid cancer), MTC, MEN2A, and MEN2B. Consequently, RET is referred to as the one implicated in numerous disorders [6, 7]. RET proto-oncogene is known as a molecular therapeutic target in thyroid cancer. Numerous factors, including as sex, age, tumor stage, and tumor grade can influence the prognosis. Therefore, the average survival rate for patients with thyroid gland cancers (95 percent) is approximately 10 years. Patients with regional and metastatic illness stages are estimated to have an overall survival rate of 75%, according to estimates. When a patient is diagnosed with distant metastasis, the prognosis is poor, with a 10-year survival rate of only 40% [8, 9]. Extra thyroidal metastasis and stage upon diagnosis are the only independent predictors of MTC patients' life expectancy. In other words, those detected at an early stage and patients without detectable recurrence had a life expectancy [10]. Postoperative calcitonin level and tumor extension have also been identified as significant prognostic variables for identifying MTC patients at high risk for disease recurrence [11]. We proposed that RET genetic mutations may be different in distinct populations. Therefore, in our recent study we found a geographical pattern of RET mutations in different populations [12].

This chapter is a summary of the current understanding of RET mutations and the most advanced therapeutic methods for RET-dependent thyroid tumors. We will discuss oncogenic RET signaling, RET inhibitors, and the major RET mutations found in MTC, as well as the necessity of RET genetic screening for the early diagnosis of MTC patients, in accordance with American Thyroid Association guidelines and genotype-phenotype correlation.

1.1 *RET* protein kinase structure and activation mechanism

RET is predominantly expressed in peripheral enteric, sympathetic, and sensory neurons, in addition to central motor, dopamine, and noradrenaline neurons. It is also expressed in branching ureteric buds and differentiating spermatogenia during embryogenesis [13]. RET contains three distinct transcripts, each of which encodes RET isoforms. RET exon 19 is present in all transcripts; however, the 3' end of exon 19 undergoes variable splicing, resulting in transcripts in which exon 19 is unspliced, spliced to exon 20, or spliced to exon 21. These transcripts encode RET isoforms with 9 (RET9), 51 (RET51), or 43 (RET43) amino acid c-terminal ends. RET9 and RET51, composed of 1072 and 1114 amino acids, are the predominant isoforms *in vivo*. These two isoforms are co-expressed in the majority of tissues but have differential developmental roles and gene expression profiles, suggesting possible discrepancies in cell-cell contact pathway regulation [14].

Tyrosine (Y1062), the last amino acid shared by all three isoforms, is phosphorylated during RET activation. Thus, alternate splicing inserts Y1062 in distinct contexts of amino acids in the three RET isoforms, imparting distinct binding potentials. An N-terminal extracellular portion of RET contains a ligand-binding domain, a cadherin ($Ca2+$-dependent cell adhesion)-like domain, and a cysteine-rich domain (near the cell membrane). This domain is a ligand for glial cell-derived neurotropic factor (GDNF), an activator protein [15]. A hydrophobic transmembrane domain and an intracellular TK domain are the other two domains. The TK domain contains several tyrosine residues (16 in RET9 and 18 in RET51), two of which are unique to RET51 at locations 1019 and 1051. The transmembrane domain ensures the close proximity of RET monomers via noncovalent interactions between receptors. Two TK subdomains, which are phosphorylated upon receptor activation and are important in the activation of intracellular signaling pathways, are present in the intracellular region [16, 17].

GDNF, NRTN, ARTN, and PSPN are ligands of the RET receptor TK that belong to GFLs. RET is unphosphorylated and inactive in the absence of these ligands. Multiple signaling pathways are activated as a result of the activation of receptor dimerization and autophosphorylation caused by the binding of ligand to the extracellular domain of the RET receptor by GFR co-receptors [18]. In other words, after GFL binds to the RET receptor, an intracytoplasmic domain within the upstream portion of RET is autophosphorylated, stabilizing the protein and necessitating subsequent downstream activity of the RET autophosphorylation cascade. In fact, phosphorylation of Tyr981, in addition to Tyr1015, Tyr1062, and Tyr1096, is crucial for beginning intracellular signal transduction cascades [19]. It is believed that RET signaling provides growth and survival signals through the RAF-MEK-ERK and PI3K-AKT-mTOR pathways [20, 21].

1.2 Intracellular signaling pathway of RET mutations

The RET gene is located on chromosome 10q11.2, is approximately 55,000 base pairs in length, includes 21 exons, and encodes a single-pass transmembrane receptor tyrosine kinase (RTK) that is mostly expressed in neural crest and urogenital tract precursor cells [10, 22]. The RET proto-oncogene encodes a receptor tyrosine kinase with four cadherin-related motifs and a cysteine-rich region in the extracellular domain, and its four ligands mentioned above. When these neurotrophic factors are administered, they activate a unique receptor system that consists of the GFR1–4 coreceptor, which is the receptor for the ligand-binding component, and the GFR2–4 coreceptor, which is responsible for the signaling component [19, 23].

Alternate 3'-spicing generates three splicing variants of RET, including RET9, RET43, and RET51. Of these, RET9 and RET51 have the most significant isoforms, each with 1072 amino acids. Through the GFR1–4 (GDNF family receptors 1–4), GFL activation of RET can be induced. These ligands activate intrinsic tyrosine kinase activity when they interact with GFR1–4 [20, 23]. In order to activate RET, the ligand must first form a complex with the necessary co-receptor. This co-receptor then interacts on the cell membrane with the RET protein, which leads to the dimerization of the receptor and the beginning of intracellular signaling via the tyrosine kinase domains [24].

Oncogenic RET proteins activate a complex network of signal transduction pathways that contributes to cellular transformation. Binding of the ligand GFR complex to RET triggers its homo dimerization, phosphorylation of tyrosine residues and subsequent intracellular signaling; subsequently, RET activation leads to increased proliferation through a complex network of second messengers, and the molecular partners and/or targets include Jun N-terminal kinase (JNK); mammalian target of rapamycin (m-TOR); phosphatidyl- inositol 3 kinase (PI3K), son of seven less (SOS); vascular endothelial growth factor (VEGF); growth actor receptor bound protein 2 (GRB2), hypoxia inducible factor 1a (HIF1a), extracellular signal-regulated kinase

(ERK), protein kinase C (PKC), pyruvate dehydrogenase kinase (PDK), phospholipase Cγ (PLCγ) [24].

The intracellular domain of RET contains autophosphorylation sites, and phosphorylated tyrosine serve as docking sites for signaling molecules [25, 26]. Phosphorylated tyrosine 1062, also known as Y1062, is one of these residues. It serves as a binding site for several different adaptor proteins, including Shc, FRS2, Dok1/4/5, IRS1/2, and Enigma, and it is critical to the capacity of mutant RET to transform cells. In addition, it was discovered that tyrosine 905 binds to Grb7/10, tyrosine 981 binds to Src, tyrosine 1015 binds to phospholipase Cγ (PLCγ), and tyrosine 1096 binds to Grb2; all of these findings were independently confirmed by other researchers [27]. Interestingly, RAS/ERK, (PI3K)/AKT, p38MAPK, and JNK pathways are activated mainly through tyrosine 1062. When the adaptor protein Shc binds to phosphorylated tyrosine 1062, it recruits the Grb2-Gab1 and Grb2-Sos complexes that then activate the PI3K/AKT and RASERK pathways, respectively (**Figure 1**) [23, 28].

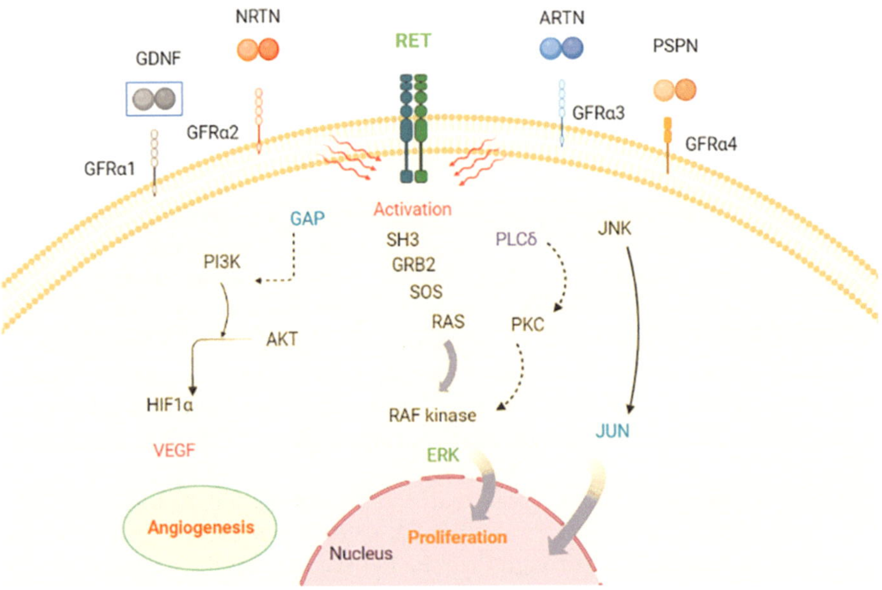

Figure 1.
RET Intracellular signaling pathway. homodimeric GFLs activate the transmembrane RET tyrosine kinase by binding to different GFR receptors; binding of the ligand GFRα complex to RET initiate the homodimerization, phosphorylation of tyrosine residues and subsequent intracellular signaling. RET activation leads to high proliferation through a complex-network of second and third messengers that is developmentally-dependent and tissue-specific.

1.3 Oncogenic RET inhibitors

Preclinical models and early phase clinical trials have explored targeted therapy through inhibition of RET and downstream signaling pathways. Phase III trials of the multi kinase inhibitors Vandetanib and Cabozantinib showed improvement in PFS (progression-free survival) but with many adverse events, which led to a trial of lower- dose Vandetanib [29].

In recent years, selective RET inhibitors have been created in an effort to obtain increased potency while also achieving lower toxicity (**Figure 2**). Pralsetinib (BLU-667) and Selpercatinib (LOXO-292) are examples of such next-generation small molecule inhibitors that have been rapidly developed and introduced into clinical testing. Both inhibitors are capable of blocking a wide spectrum of RET changes, including M918T, C634W, gatekeeper mutations V804L and V804M, KIF5B-RET, and CCDC6-RET, according to the functional tests that were conducted utilising a variety of in vitro and in vivo models. It is important to note that LOXO-292 and BLU-667 have substantially less activity against VEGFR2 in comparison to modifications in RET, which could potentially reduce their toxicity [30].

The RET receptor can be inhibited effectively and selectively by LOXO-292. Both RET mutations, as observed in MTC, and RET fusions are the targets of this medication (seen in PTC, PDTC, and ATC). The RET V804 gatekeeper mutation, which is linked to resistance to RET-targeted kinase inhibitors, was the primary focus of the research that went into the development of this medication. Because LOXO-292 is able to pass the blood-brain barrier and achieve therapeutic concentrations in the central nervous system, it has the potential to be used as a therapy for brain metastases caused by RET mutation or fusion. At the annual meeting of the American Society of Clinical Oncology in 2018, preliminary findings from the LIBRETTO-001 phase 1 dose escalation and expansion trial were presented. Fatigue ranging from grade 1 to 2, diarrhea, constipation, dry mouth, nausea, and dyspnea were the side effects that occurred the most frequently (10 percent to 20 percent). Asymptomatic increase of the alanine aminotransferase level and a case of tumor lysis syndrome were the two conditions in question here. The maximum dose that the patient could tolerate was not achieved. The LIBRETTO-001 clinical trial is currently in the expansion phase, during which additional patients with RET-mutated MTC and RET-fusion malignancies, such as PTC (papillary thyroid cancer), PDTC (poorly differentiated thyroid cancer), and ATC (anaplastic thyroid cancer), are being enrolled.

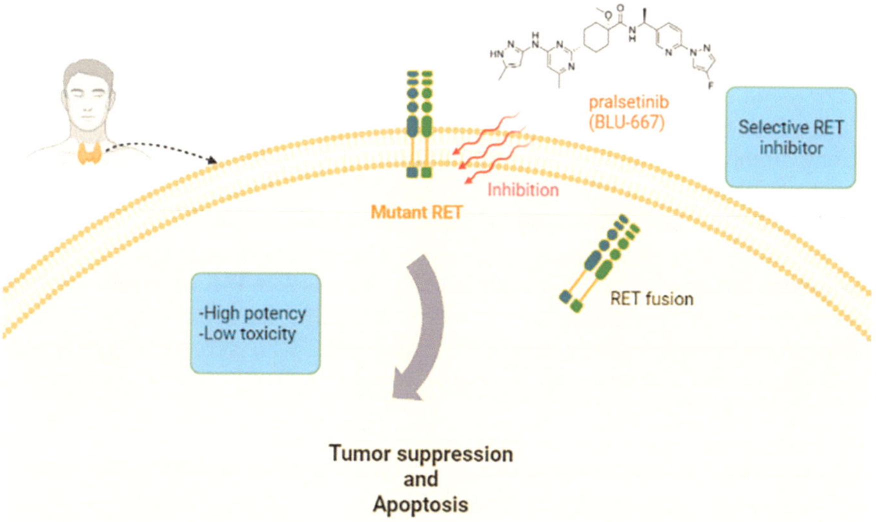

Figure 2.
Oncogenic RET signaling and selective RET inhibitors

Additionally, BLU-292 is an extremely selective and highly effective RET inhibitor. It works in a manner very similar to that of LOXO-292, in that it targets RET fusions as well as RET mutations, such as the RET V804 mutation. A phase 1 escalation/expansion clinical trial of BLU-667 is currently being conducted, and the results of the trial were reported at the annual meeting of the American Association for Cancer Research in 2018. This study's objectives include determining the maximum tolerated dose, assessing safety, analyzing pharmacokinetics, and evaluating preliminary anti-cancer activity. Constipation, elevated alanine aminotransferase and aspartate amino-transferase, hypertension, leukopenia, headache, sleeplessness, and exhaustion were the only side effects of the low toxicity that was seen [31].

BOS172738, TPX- 0046, and TAS0953/HM06 are likewise in the early phases of development as selective RET inhibitors. In addition to the RET V804M gatekeeper mutation, multiple alternative pathways of acquired resistance to MKIs have been described. Mechanisms of resistance to selective RET remain a major field of study. According to a preclinical investigation, the unique solvent front mutation KIF5B-RET G810R may develop on-target resistance to Selpercatinib and Pralsetinib, however it remains vulnerable to TPX-0046, a selective RET inhibitor built with a macrocyclic structure to target active RET confirmation [30].

In conclusion, over the past three decades, the involvement of RET activating mutations and rearrangements in carcinogenesis has been proven. With the emergence of extremely selective RET inhibitors, there is significant enthusiasm in the RET sector. In preliminary phase I/II trials, the next-generation selective RET inhibitors Selpercatinib and Pralsetib displayed excellent clinical efficacy and safety. Both agents have obtained breakthrough designations from the FDA. Unanswered questions include the PFS, DOR (duration of response), and OS (overall survival) with these drugs; if all RET aberrant tumors respond similarly for a tissue-agnostic indication; and the mechanisms of acquired resistance to the potent RET inhibitors. In addition, combination therapies that investigate the simultaneous inhibition of RET and associated pathways will shed light on the clinical efficacy of such techniques [30].

According to clinical and preclinical studies, initiation of RET kinase activity has been characterized as a target for a number of tyrosine kinase inhibitors [32]. The finding of molecular targets in thyroid cancer has led to the development of treatments for patients who have advanced forms of the disease. These treatments include FDA-approved drugs such as Cabozantinib and Vandetanib for MTC and Sorafenib and Lenvatinib for differentiated thyroid cancer [33, 34].

Strong inhibition of the target proteins VEGFR-2, MET, RET, KIT, AXL, and TIE2 is provided by Cabozantinib. Because of its potent ability to inhibit RET; Cabozantinib was identified as a particularly promising candidate for treatment in MTC patients. Cabozantinib, in contrast to Vandetanib, does not reduce EGFR activity to a significant degree. Other tyrosine kinase receptor inhibitors, such as ZD6474, which are medicines that are active when taken orally, have an effect on VEGFR-2 and limit the actions of RET tyrosine kinase. In patients with metastatic familial MTC who were participating in a clinical research, it was revealed that ZD6474 therapy triggered some degree of cure [12].

1.4 *RET* proto-oncogene mutations

There have been a total of 100 different mutations found in the RET gene so far, and with the exception of a few that cause dual phenotypes, the majority of them can be classified as either having a loss of function or a gain of function. Gain-of-function mutations in RET are primarily what cause RET-related malignancies, and these mutations may be broken down into two categories: those that modify cysteine residues in the cysteine-rich domain, and those that alter residues in the RET-KD. Within the first group, the mutated residue that occurs most frequently in MEN2A patients is Cys634. This occurs because the removal of one-half of an intra-molecular disulfide bond makes it possible to form an intermolecular disulfide bond with a second mutant molecule. This results in constitutive receptor dimerization and aberrant signaling. It is not known if activating mutations within RET-KD directly lead to constitutive dimer formation or whether the mechanism for activating mutations is more diverse. RET transformation can be produced by a wide variety of mutations, including L790F, Y791F, S891A, and R844L, but the resulting symptoms are only moderately severe MTC and MEN2A. In contrast, the M918T mutation has a very high capacity for transformation and is present in 95% of MEN2B patients. This mutation is responsible for the disease. A number of mucosal, ophthalmic, and skeletal disorders are included in the MEN2B phenotype. In addition to the thyroid and adrenal glands, this phenotype affects the skeleton. In stark contrast to the MEN2A dimerizing mutations, in which Tyr905 is necessary for oncogenesis, the M918T RET mutation does not require this residue in order to become activated [35]. This implies that various underlying mechanisms disrupt RET activation's normal control in MEN2A and MEN2B. Furthermore, M918T RET specifically targets novel substrates like STAT3 that may aid in cell transformation [36]. In addition to transforming mutations that occur inside intact RET, chromosome translocations have the potential to produce oncogenic fusions that include the RET kinase domain (RET/PTC oncogenes). These oncogenes are responsible for the development of PTC. RET/PTC fusion proteins are found in the cytoplasm and contain RET-KD from the beginning of exon 12 (which begins at Glu713) all the way through the C terminus. The N-terminal domain of RET/PTC is often a dimerization domain derived from the fusion partner in many instances. Notably, reducing the converting potential of RET/PTC by mutating the residue that corresponds to Tyr905 in wild-type RET results in less transformation [37, 38].

As previously mentioned, RET missense mutations in the germline are linked to MEN2A, MEN2B, and FMTC, whereas sporadic MTC is thought to result from a somatic mutation in the tumor cells, RET mutations are primarily missense and located in exons 10, 11, 13, 14, 15, and 16 (RET's extracellular domain) (in the TK domain) [5, 39, 40]. A ligand-independent dimerization of receptor molecules, increased phosphorylation of intracellular substrates, and cell transformation can be caused by a mutation of the extracellular cysteine in codon 634 of exon 11 of RET. A mutation in the intracellular TK (for example, codon 918) has no effect on receptor dimerization, but it does promote constitutive activation of intracellular signaling pathways, which in turn culminates in cellular transformation [21, 41].

Exons 10 and 11 have the FMTC-specific mutations as well. Exon 8 (codons 532 and 533), exon 13, (codons 768, 790, and 791), (codons 804 and 844), (codon 891), and exon 16 have also been shown to have non-cysteine point mutations (codon 912) [42]. According to a recent meta-analysis, 39 distinct RET germline mutations have been discovered in FMTC patients from various families since 1993. All mutations were missense type and dispersed among exons 5, 8, 10, 11, 13, 14, 15, and 16 with the exception of a 9-bp duplication (after codon 531, exon 8). In FMTC, age-specific penetrance of cancer growth and nodal metastasis were strongly linked with particular germline RET mutations [43]. Overall, mutations in codons 609, 611, 618, and 620 of exon 10, codon 768 of exon 13, and codon 804 of exon 14 are most frequently related with FMTC. When FMTC is related with mutations in codon 634 of exon 11, C634R is nearly never observed, while C634Y is the most prevalent variant [21].

1.5 Germline screening of RET mutations

The genetic testing for RET germline mutation has demonstrated 100 percent sensitivity and specificity in identifying persons at risk for developing MTC. In comparison to the current standard of annual biochemical monitoring, such as blood calcitonin, this genetic assay allows for earlier and more conclusive diagnosis and clinical management of people who have a familial risk for MTC. Once a person is identified as having a RET mutation, they must receive thorough counseling. In order to give a preventive thyroidectomy to asymptomatic individuals who are diagnosed as RET mutation carriers, it is necessary to identify and test at-risk family members [4].

Since prophylactic thyroidectomy can prevent hMTC, the American Thyroid Association suggests that all patients with MTC be offered germline RET testing [44]. Based on a model that categorizes mutations into risk levels using genotype-phenotype correlations, recommendations for the scheduling of prophylactic thyroidectomy and the extent of surgical resection are made (A-D). The highest risk of MTC is associated with ATA level D (ATA-D) mutations. Codons 883 (exon 15) and 918 (exon 16) are two of these mutations that are linked to the lowest age of onset, the highest risk of metastasis, and the highest fatality rate. A lower but still significant prevalence of aggressive MTC is linked to ATA level C (ATA-C) mutations, which include codon 634 changes (exon 11). ATA-B mutations, which include mutations at codons 609, 611, 618, 620 (exon 10) and 630, are associated with a decreased risk for severe MTC mutations (exon 11). ATA-A mutations are associated with the "least severe" risk. When they have preventative thyroidectomy at age 4 years, these patients have lower serum calcitonin levels, a lower tumor stage, and a better rate of biochemical cure compared to ATA-B mutation carriers of the same age [45]. RET mutations can be found at codons 768, 790, 791 (exon 13), 804 (exon 14), and 891 in ATA-A mutations (exon 15). ATA made the decision to develop specialized MTC Clinical Guidelines in order to compile and update the vast amount of MTC-related literature, as well as to integrate this information with evidence-based medicine and the feedback of a panel of experienced physicians [21, 46].

There are limited reports of these mutations in Iranian families with MTC in the literature [47, 48]. In our recent study, we tested individuals with MTC and their MTC-affected first-degree relatives for RET exon10 mutations. In our latest investigation, 14 individuals with sMTC and FMTC were found to have six distinct mutations in exon10 of RET that were confined to codons 611, 618, and 620, but not codon 609. This data revealed an atypical distribution of RET exon10 mutations in comparison to other groups. In our study population, exon10 of the RET proto-oncogene was mutation-free in MEN2A, MEN2B, and pheochromocytoma. However, exon10 mutations in MEN2A have been found in numerous populations. C611Y and C620R were the most prevalent mutations in exon10 among patients with FMTC and sMTC, respectively [49, 50].

Codon 620 of exon 10 has generally been shown to include eight different variants, including seven missense mutations and one synonymous mutation. The codon in exon 10 with the greatest frequency of mutations during our analysis was codon 620. In other words, more over 50% of the mutations in our investigation were caused by codon 620. Additionally, neither synonymous nor nonsense mutations in exon 10 of the RET proto-oncogene were found in our study population. None of the cysteine codons in exon 10 had any mutations. The findings of this study suggest that mutations in exon 10 of the RET proto-oncogene are limited to three critical cysteine codons (611, 618, and 620), which were only identified in Iranian patients with FMTC and likely sMTC. All patients with exon 10 mutations, with the exception of one, had the haplotype G691S/S904S. In the current analysis, no mutation in the RET proto-exon oncogene's 10 in the syndromic type of MTC was found [50].

Since the research of other exons within the same gene has received less attention, we investigated the incidence of germ line mutations in exon 2 of the RET proto-oncogene in Iranian patients with MTC. The RET gene has the nucleotide substitutions c135G>A/A45A (rs1800858) in exon 2 and c.337+9G>A (rs2435351) and c.337+137G>T (rs2505530) in the intronic region. Among patients and relatives, the genotype and allele frequencies with the highest and lowest frequencies, respectively, were c.337+137G>T (rs2505530) and c135G>A/A45A (rs1800858). Also, no link was found between identified nucleotide alterations and disease phenotype, gender, or race. No mutations resulting in altered amino acid sequences in exon 2 or exon-intron splice sites were identified. However, additional research is advised to determine the likely correlation between discovered variants and the presence or absences of other mutations in other RET major exons, as well as to determine the haplotype association with the disease [51].

217 people were included in order to study the spectrum of prominent RET germline mutations in exons 10, 11, and 16 in hereditary MTC in the Iranian population. Leukocytes' genomic DNAs were isolated utilizing the Salting Out/Proteinase K technique. The mutations were detected using PCR-RFLP and DNA sequencing. In 217 subjects, 43 missense mutations were found in exons 10, 11, and 16 (6 percent, 13 percent, and 16 percent, respectively) (0.9 percent). In addition, a new germline mutation was found in exon 11 (S686N). In addition, eight individuals had four distinct SNPs in intron 16. The data revealed the frequency profile of RET mutations in Iranian patients with MTC (19.8 percent). In our population, C634G was the most prevalent mutation, but in most populations it was C634R. Collectively, these data highlight the significance of the genetic background of family members of any MTC patient [5].

Finally, it is advised that other RET exons, particularly those with a high frequency of mutations, such as exons 13, 14, and 15, be studied. Additionally, direct sequencing analysis is a reliable tool for detecting unknown RETS mutations. In addition, the transformative activity and functional effect(s) of novel RET mutations such as S686N and intronic polymorphisms have yet to be determined (**Figure 3**) [5].

1.6 The relationship between RET tyrosine kinase inhibition and MTC treatment

Recent RET-kinase inhibitors for the treatment of MTC are through various levels of preclinical and clinical testing [52]. A group has launched a phase II clinical research assessing the efficacy of oral ZD6474 (Zactima®) in patients with locally advanced or metastatic MTC: of the 20 patients accrued to date, around 30% have seen objective remissions. Other inhibitors of RET activity targeting various areas of its molecular biology and signaling pathway are in development [24, 53, 54]. The most important drugs for MTC treatment is listed in **Figure 4**.

Patients with MTC are evaluated using tumor markers (calcitonin and carcinoembryonic antigen; CEA), a complete and precise ultrasonography of the neck, and genetic testing. Cross-sectional imaging may be obtained for surgical planning or when suspected distant metastases are present. Biochemical testing is required to exclude primary hyperparathyroidism and PHEO (pheochromocytoma). After this, a total thyroidectomy with central neck dissection is often advised, and in rare instances, more extensive surgery may be required (if indicated by the preoperative

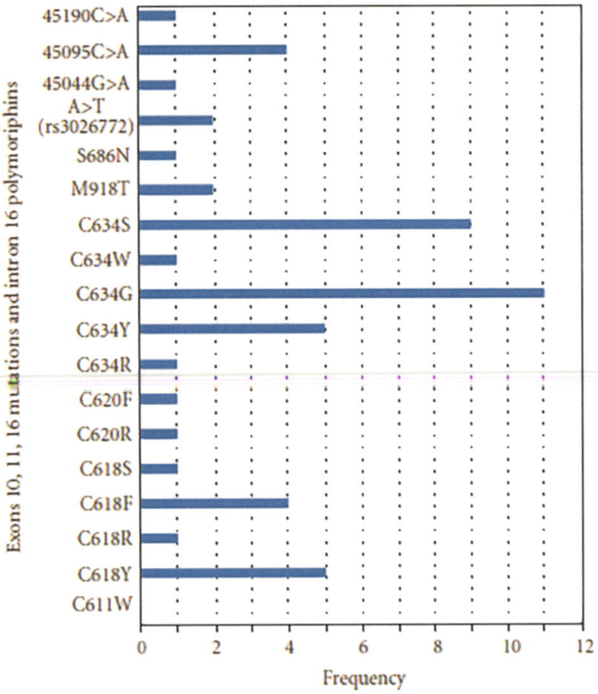

Figure 3.
The allele frequency of the RET proto-oncogene mutations in Iranian patients with MTC.

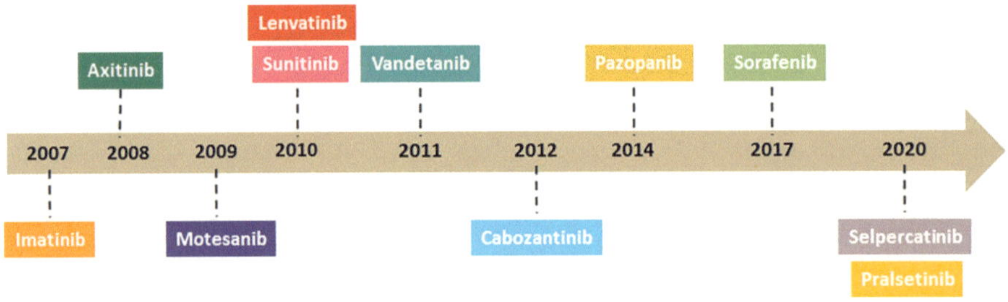

Figure 4.
The most important FDA-approved drugs for MTC according to their approved years or current phases of clinical trials.

assessment). External beam radiation therapy may improve loco regional control if the patient has a high risk of recurrence [34]. Since the response to first therapy influences survival and recurrence risk, an experienced multidisciplinary team should be included from the start [55]. Many of these concerns are addressed in the new American Thyroid Association (ATA) guidelines for MTC management [56].

Watchful waiting, surgery, radiation, cryo ablation, and chemoembolization are treatment options for asymptomatic residual, recurrent, and distant metastatic disease in MTC and differentiated thyroid carcinoma (DTC). In order to minimize skeletal-related occurrences in MTC patients, receptor activator of nuclear factor kappa B ligand (RANKL) inhibitors or intravenous bisphosphonate are often administered [12, 57].

2. ATA Recommendations for MTC management

Since hMTC can be prevented by prophylactic thyroidectomy, the American Thyroid Association (ATA) suggests that all patients with MTC should be offered germline RET mutation testing for mutation discovery and improved patient and family treatment (particularly in RET-positive cases) [44, 56]. Nevertheless, the updated ATA has altered the existing risk categories for hMTC. It is now recommended to undertake genotype to phenotype correlation of disease in order to identify mutations that enhance the risk levels of patients with MTC, hence determining the necessity of prophylactic thyroidectomy and the extent of surgical resection.

Recommendations for the scheduling of prophylactic thyroidectomy and surgical area resection are derived on genotype-phenotype correlations used to categorize mutation risk levels. The preceding ATA advice categorized risk based on four mutation levels: A, B, C, and D. ATA-D mutations, especially codons 883 (exon 15) and 918 (exon 16), were related with the lowest age of onset, the greatest incidence of metastasis, and the highest fatality rate. In the most recent amended ATA guideline, a new "highest risk" (HST) category has been created, which covers patients with MEN2B and the RET codon M918T mutation [46].

ATA-C mutations, including mutations at codon 634 (exon 11), were assumed to provide a decreased risk of aggressive MTC. This category has been renamed "high risk" (H) in the new ATA guideline and now covers patients with MEN2A and RET codon C634 mutations. ATA-B mutations, including mutations at codons 609, 611, 618, 620 (exon 10) and 630, carry a decreased risk for severe MTC mutations (exon 11). ATA-A mutations are associated with the lowest risk. When they have preventive thyroidectomy at age 4 years, these patients have lower serum calcitonin levels, a lower tumor stage, and a better rate of biochemical cure compared to ATA-B mutation carriers of the same age. RET mutations at codons 768, 790, 791 (exon 13), 804 (exon 14), and 891 (exon 15) are seen in ATA-A mutations. The revised ATA guideline combines the current A and B levels into a new category, "moderate risk" (MOD), which includes patients with hMTC and RET codon mutations other than M918T and C634 (**Tables 1** and **2**) [12, 58].

Mutation location	Exon	Mutation	Phenotype	Mutation risk level according to 2009ATA
Extra cellular cadherin like domain	5	G321R	FMTC/MEN2A	A
Extra cellular cysteine rich domain	8	C515S	FMTC/MEN2A	A
		532 duplication	FMTC	A
		529/531	FMTC	?
		G533C	FMTC/MEN2A	A
		532 duplication	FMTC	A
		531/9bp duplication	FMTC/MEN2A	A
	10	R600Q	FMTC/MEN2A	A
		K603E	FMTC/MEN2A	A
		K603Q	FMTC	A

Mutation location	Exon	Mutation	Phenotype	Mutation risk level according to 2009ATA
		Y606C	FMTC	A
		C609F/R/G/S/Y	FMTC/MEN2A/HSCR	B
		C611R/G/F/S/W/Y	FMTC/MEN2A/HSCR	B
		C618R/G/F/S/Y	FMTC/MEN2A/HSCR	B
		C620R/G/F/S/W/Y	FMTC/MEN2A/HSCR	B
		C630R/F/S/Y	FMTC/MEN2A	B
	11	D631Y	FMTC	B
		633	MEN2A	?
		633/9bp duplication	FMTC/MEN2A	B
		634/12bp duplication	FMTC/MEN2A	B
		C634R	MEN2A/CLA	C
		C634G/F/S/W/Y	FMTC/MEN2A/CLA	C
		634/12bp duplication	MEN2A	B
		635/insertion ELCR/ T636P	FMTC/MEN2A	A
		637	MEN2A	?
		S649L	FMTC/MEN2A	A
		K666E	FMTC/MEN2A	A
	13	E768D	FMTC/MEN2A/ sMTC	A
		N777S	FMTC	A
		778	FMTC	?
		N776S	FMTC/MEN2A	A
		781	FMTC	?
		L790F	FMTC/MEN2A	A
		Y791F	FMTC/MEN2A	A
	14	V804L	FMTC/MEN2A	A
		V804M	FMTC/MEN2A/ sMTC	A
		V804M+E805K	MEN2B	D
		V804M+Y806C	MEN2B	D
		G819K	FMTC	A
		R833C	FMTC/ MEN2B	A
		R844Q	FMTC/ MEN2B	A
		V804M/E805K	MEN 2B	D
		V804M/Y806C	MEN 2B	D
		804/844	FMTC	?
		852	FMTC	?

Mutation location	Exon	Mutation	Phenotype	Mutation risk level according to 2009ATA
Intra cellular tyrosine kinase domain	15	R866W	FMTC/MEN2A	A
		876	FMTC	?
		A883F	MEN2B/ sMTC	D
		S891A	FMTC/MEN2A	A
	16	R912P	FMTC/MEN2A/ MEN2B	A
		M918T	sMTC/MEN2B	D
		920	sMTC/MEN2B	D
		922	sMTC/MEN2B	D
	13/14	V804M+V778I	FMTC/MEN2A	B
	14/15	V804M+S904C	MEN2B/ MEN2A	D
	13/16	768/919	FMTC	?
	14/15	V804M/S904C	MEN 2B	D

Table 1.
Genotype-phenotype correlations and risk levels for different populations of aggressive MTC according to ATA.

Family/ patient No.	MTC age of onset	Gender	Exon	Codon	Nucleotide/amino acid (RET Mutation)	Phenotype
2	26	F	11	634	TGC → TAC (Cys634Tyr)	MEN2A
5	10	M	14	804	GTG → ATG (Val804Met)	Sporadic
6	31	F	10	611	TGC → TAC (Cys611Tyr)	Sporadic
7	13	F	11	634	TGC → CGC (Cys634Arg)	Sporadic
11	27	F	10	618	TGC → CGC (Cys618Arg)	Sporadic
21	15	F	11	634	TGC → CGC (Cys634Arg)	Sporadic
26	26	M	11	630	TGC → CGC (Cys630Arg)	FMTC
31/1	21	F	11	634	TGC → CGC (Cys634Arg)	Sporadic
31/2	21	F	11	634	TGC → CGC (Cys634Arg)	MEN2A
31/3	21	M	11	634	TGC → CGC (Cys634Arg)	Sporadic
39	20	M	11	634	TGC → CGC (Cys634Arg)	Sporadic
51	22	M	11	634	TGC → CGC (Cys634Arg)	Sporadic
53	14	F	16	918	ATG → ACG (Met918Thr)	MEN2B

Table 2.
Correlation between the genetic findings and the phenotype of the respective Iranian population.

3. Geographical pattern of *RET* mutations in various populations

This phenomenon, known as allelic heterogeneity, occurs when different mutations at the same locus result in the same phenotype. A diverse mutation pattern has been identified in this gene as a result of the characterization of multiple RET proto-oncogene mutations. It suggests that these mutations in distinct populations are related with a slightly diverse phenotype in various countries. Despite the identification of codon 634 of the RET proto-oncogene as a hot spot codon in the evolution of MEN2A and FMTC, the amino acid alteration at this codon is almost unique to each group. The identification of RET mutations in MTC patients was examined extensively in a number of diverse groups, which are briefly summarized in this section (**Table 3**) [59].

Population	RET mutation	Reference
American	The V804M mutation was observed in MEN2A patients frequently, rather than many other populations in which the cysteine codons have mutated.	[60, 61]
Australian	The most frequent variants were V804L, V804M, and C634R in MEN2A patients. Furthermore, the C620R, C634Y, and C634R were found in higher incidence in FMTC cases.	[62, 63]
Brazilian, Chinese, Indian and Moroccan	The C634R and the C634Y were the most common mutations in MEN2A patients, respectively. Also in Brazilian FMTCs the G533C was observed frequently. This mutation is known as a rare mutation in many other countries.	[64–68]
Czech Republic	The C634R mutation in MEN2A patients and V804M and Y791F mutations in FMTC patients were the most had the most common occurrence.	[69]
French	The C634Y and C634R mutations in MEN2A, and the C618S and C620R mutations in FMTC were the most frequent.	[70–72]
Germany	The C634R and C620F mutations in MEN2A, and the E768D mutation in FMTC were more prevalent in comparison with other mutations	[58, 73]
Greek	The G533C mutation in exon eight of the RET gene was observed in FMTC and sMTC patients with high prevalence. In addition, K-RAS and BRAF gene mutations in a Greek cohort of sporadic PTC and MTC carcinomas are reported.	[74–76]
Iranian	The C634Y and then the C634R mutations were observed MEN2A patients with the highest frequencies. In addition, the C634Y, C634W, and C630Y mutations were the most common in FMTC. In sMTC individuals, the C634R mutation occurred with the highest frequency. Interestingly, there was not any mutation in MTC patients in hot spot codon 609 (exon10) in this population.	[5, 47, 48, 50, 77–79]
Italian	The most common mutations in MEN2A were C634R, C618R, and C634Y, respectively, and in sMTC were V804M, E768D, and S891A.	[80, 81]
Japanese	The C620Y, C634R, and C634S were frequent mutations in MEN2A patients. Also in FMTC the C618Y and C630S mutations had higher incidence.	[82]
Korean	The C634Y, C634R, and C618R were the most common mutations in MEN2A. In addition, FMTC patients in this population had high C618S mutation frequency.	[83–85]
Mexican	The C634Y mutation was higher in MEN2A patients than the other mutations.	[83]

Population	RET mutation	Reference
Portuguese	The C634R and C611Y mutations in MEN2A, and the C634R and C634Y mutations in FMTC were common. Moreover, in sMTC the V804M, L760F, and C620R mutations were observed in most of the cases Recently, two novel mutations (C515W and T636M) associated with MTC have been also identified in this population.	[2, 86–88]
South Africa	The C634S mutation had the highest frequency in MEN2A patients.	[89–91]
Spanish	The most common mutations were C634R and then C634Y in MEN2A patients, while the C634R mutation in FMTC had a higher frequency. Interestingly, the predominant mutation in MEN2B cases in all evaluated populations was M918T in exon 16 of the RET proto oncogene.	[92–95]

Table 3.
RET mutational spectrum in different populations.

4. Conclusion

RET mutations do not simply determine MTC formation. These cancers likely carry mutations in additional genes, and it may be necessary to be aware of these mutations in order to consider combination therapy. This may provide new targets for the combination of RET inhibitors with other drugs that target these pathways [7]. Although a number of patients with refractory MTC have been treated with a variety of TKIs over the past few years, it is still unclear if the RET genotype of tumor cells influences clinical response to these medications [38, 54].

The thyroid cancer is the most prevalent endocrine cancer. In terms of diagnosis and preventive treatment, MTC has the strongest hereditary component among other kinds of thyroid cancer, according to ATA standards. MEN2B RET proto-oncogene mutations appear to be predominantly fixed at the M918T location in exon 16. However, mutations associated with MEN2A and FMTC vary amongst populations. For diagnosis, it will be important to evaluate and identify population-specific trends in point mutations [12]. Although there are several approaches in the treatment of RET-associated cancers; including monoclonal antibodies, kinase inhibitors, adaptor-protein binding inhibitors, dimerization inhibitors and gene therapy. Searching for specific inhibitors of RET kinase is a promising strategy. Indeed, reagents such as antioxidants, which abrogate RET dimerization, may also be useful in the treatment of MTC and PTC. Moreover, recent advances in RNA interference technology are providing a novel tool for cancer therapy [23].

More research is required and comprehensive clinical studies must be undertaken, but the preliminary findings are encouraging and optimistic. In the fight against cancer, the in-depth study of cancer and the identification of solid therapeutic targets and effective pharmacological agents have once again proven fruitful.

Author details

Shabnam Heydarzadeh[1,2] and Mehdi Hedayati[2*]

1 Department of Biochemistry, School of Biological Sciences, Falavarjan Branch Islamic Azad University, Isfahan, Iran

2 Cellular and Molecular Endocrine Research Center, Research Institute for Endocrine Sciences, Shahid Beheshti University of Medical Sciences, Tehran, Iran

*Address all correspondence to: hedayati@endocrine.ac.ir; hedayati47@gmail.com

References

[1] Dvořáková Š, Vaclavikova E, Sýkorová V, Dušková J, Vlček P, Ryška A, et al. New multiple somatic mutations in the RET proto-oncogene associated with a sporadic medullary thyroid carcinoma. Thyroid. 2006;**16**(3):311-316

[2] Moura MM, Cavaco BM, Pinto AE, Domingues R, Santos JR, Cid MO, et al. Correlation of RET somatic mutations with clinicopathological features in sporadic medullary thyroid carcinomas. British Journal of Cancer. 2009;**100**(11): 1777-1783

[3] Elisei R, Cosci B, Romei C, Bottici V, Renzini G, Molinaro E, et al. Prognostic significance of somatic RET oncogene mutations in sporadic medullary thyroid cancer: a 10-year follow-up study. The Journal of Clinical Endocrinology and Metabolism. 2008;**93**(3):682-687

[4] Sippel RS, Kunnimalaiyaan M, Chen H. Current management of medullary thyroid cancer. The Oncologist. 2008;**13**(5):539-547

[5] Hedayati M, Zarif Yeganeh M, Sheikhol Eslami S, Rezghi Barez S, Hoghooghi Rad L, Azizi F. Predominant RET germline mutations in exons 10, 11, and 16 in Iranian patients with hereditary medullary thyroid carcinoma. Journal of Thyroid Research. 2011;**2011**

[6] Ibáñez CF. Structure and physiology of the RET receptor tyrosine kinase. Cold Spring Harbor Perspectives in Biology. 2013;**5**(2):a009134

[7] Prazeres H, Torres J, Rodrigues F, Couto JP, Vinagre J, Sobrinho-Simoes M, et al. How to treat a signal? Current basis for RET-genotype-oriented choice of kinase inhibitors for the treatment of medullary thyroid cancer. Journal of Thyroid Research. 2011;**2011**

[8] Agrawal N, Jiao Y, Sausen M, Leary R, Bettegowda C, Roberts NJ, et al. Exomic sequencing of medullary thyroid cancer reveals dominant and mutually exclusive oncogenic mutations in RET and RAS. The Journal of Clinical Endocrinology and Metabolism. 2013;**98**(2):E364-E369

[9] Roman S, Lin R, Sosa JA. Prognosis of medullary thyroid carcinoma: demographic, clinical, and pathologic predictors of survival in 1252 cases. Cancer: Interdisciplinary International Journal of the American Cancer Society. 2006;**107**(9):2134-2142

[10] De Groot JWB, Plukker JTM, Wolffenbuttel BHR, Wiggers T, Sluiter WJ, Links TP. Determinants of life expectancy in medullary thyroid cancer: age does not matter. Clinical Endocrinology. 2006;**65**(6):729-736

[11] Pellegriti G, Leboulleux S, Baudin E, Bellon N, Scollo C, Travagli JP, et al. Long-term outcome of medullary thyroid carcinoma in patients with normal postoperative medical imaging. British Journal of Cancer. 2003;**88**(10): 1537-1542

[12] Hedayati M, Zarif Yeganeh M, Sheikholeslami S, Afsari F. Diversity of mutations in the RET proto-oncogene and its oncogenic mechanism in medullary thyroid cancer. Critical Reviews in Clinical Laboratory Sciences. 2016;**53**(4):217-227

[13] Meng X, Lindahl M, Hyvonen ME, Parvinen M, de Rooij DG, Hess MW, et al. Regulation of cell fate decision of undifferentiated spermatogonia by GDNF. Science. 2000;**287**(5457): 1489-1493

[14] Hickey JG, Myers SM, Tian X, Zhu SJV, Shaw JL, Andrew SD, et al.

RET-mediated gene expression pattern is affected by isoform but not oncogenic mutation. Genes, Chromosomes and Cancer. 2009;**48**(5):429-440

[15] Arighi E, Borrello MG, Sariola H. RET tyrosine kinase signaling in development and cancer. Cytokine and Growth Factor Reviews. 2005;**16**(4–5): 441-467

[16] Colombo-Benkmann M, Li Z, Riemann B, Hengst K, Herbst H, Keuser R, et al. Characterization of the RET protooncogene transmembrane domain mutation S649L associated with nonaggressive medullary thyroid carcinoma. European Journal of Endocrinology. 2008;**158**(6):811-816

[17] de Groot JWB, Links TP, Plukker JTM, Lips CJM, Hofstra RMW. RET as a diagnostic and therapeutic target in sporadic and hereditary endocrine tumors. Endocrine Reviews. 2006;**27**(5):535-560

[18] Phay JE, Shah MH. Targeting RET receptor tyrosine kinase activation in cancer. Clinical Cancer Research. 2010; **16**(24):5936-5941

[19] Airaksinen MS, Saarma M. The GDNF family: Signalling, biological functions and therapeutic value. Nature Reviews Neuroscience. 2002;**3**(5): 383-394

[20] Takahashi M. The GDNF/RET signaling pathway and human diseases. Cytokine and Growth Factor Reviews. 2001;**12**(4):361-373

[21] Yeganeh MZ, Sheikholeslami S, Hedayati M. RET proto oncogene mutation detection and medullary thyroid carcinoma prevention. Asian Pacific Journal of Cancer Prevention. 2015;**16**(6):2107-2117

[22] Mitsiades N, Fagin JA. Molecular genetics of thyroid cancer: pathogenetic significance and clinical applications. In: Genetic Diagnosis of Endocrine Disorders. Elsevier; 2010. pp. 117-138

[23] Kodama Y, Asai N, Kawai K, Jijiwa M, Murakumo Y, Ichihara M, et al. The RET proto-oncogene: a molecular therapeutic target in thyroid cancer. Cancer Science. 2005;**96**(3):143-148

[24] Boikos SA, Stratakis CA. Molecular mechanisms of medullary thyroid carcinoma, current approaches in diagnosis and treatment. Histology and Histopathology. 2008

[25] Pützer BM, Drosten M. The RET proto-oncogene: a potential target for molecular cancer therapy. Trends in Molecular Medicine. 2004;**10**(7):351-357

[26] Santoro M, Melillo RM, Carlomagno F, Vecchio G, Fusco A. Minireview: RET: normal and abnormal functions. Endocrinology. 2004;**145**(12): 5448-5451

[27] Encinas M, Crowder RJ, Milbrandt J, Johnson EM. Tyrosine 981, a novel ret autophosphorylation site, binds c-Src to mediate neuronal survival. Journal of Biological Chemistry. 2004;**279**(18): 18262-18269

[28] Maeda K, Murakami H, Yoshida R, Ichihara M, Abe A, Hirai M, et al. Biochemical and biological responses induced by coupling of Gab1 to phosphatidylinositol 3-kinase in RET-expressing cells. Biochemical and Biophysical Research Communications. 2004;**323**(1):345-354

[29] Gild ML, Bullock M, Robinson BG, Clifton-Bligh R. Multikinase inhibitors: a new option for the treatment of thyroid cancer. Nature Reviews Endocrinology. 2011;**7**(10):617

[30] Subbiah V, Yang D, Velcheti V, Drilon A, Meric-Bernstam F. State-of-the-art strategies for targeting RET-dependent cancers. Journal of Clinical Oncology. 2020;**38**(11):1209

[31] Cabanillas ME, Ryder M, Jimenez C. Targeted therapy for advanced thyroid cancer: Kinase inhibitors and beyond. Endocrine Reviews. 2019;**40**(6): 1573-1604

[32] Omur O, Baran Y. An update on molecular biology of thyroid cancers. Critical Reviews in Oncology/ Hematology. 2014;**90**(3):233-252

[33] Huang L, Jiang S, Shi Y. Tyrosine kinase inhibitors for solid tumors in the past 20 years (2001–2020). Journal of Hematology and Oncology. 2020;**13**(1): 1-23

[34] Weitzman SP, Cabanillas ME. The treatment landscape in thyroid cancer: A focus on cabozantinib. Cancer Management and Research. 2015;7:265

[35] Kawamoto Y, Takeda K, Okuno Y, Yamakawa Y, Ito Y, Taguchi R, et al. Identification of RET autophosphorylation sites by mass spectrometry. Journal of Biological Chemistry. 2004;**279**(14): 14213-14224

[36] Schuringa JJ, Wojtachnio K, Hagens W, Vellenga E, Buys CHCM, Hofstra R, et al. MEN2A-RET-induced cellular transformation by activation of STAT3. Oncogene. 2001;**20**(38): 5350-5358

[37] Buckwalter TLF, Venkateswaran A, Lavender M, La Perle K, Cho J-Y, Robinson ML, et al. The roles of phosphotyrosines-294,-404, and-451 in RET/PTC1-induced thyroid tumor formation. Oncogene. 2002;**21**(53): 8166-8172

[38] Knowles PP, Murray-Rust J, Kjær S, Scott RP, Hanrahan S, Santoro M, et al. Structure and chemical inhibition of the RET tyrosine kinase domain. Journal of Biological Chemistry. 2006;**281**(44): 33577-33587

[39] Raue F, Frank-Raue K. Update multiple endocrine neoplasia type 2. Familial Cancer. 2010;**9**(3):449-457

[40] Segouffin-Cariou C, Billaud M. Transforming ability of MEN2A-RET requires activation of the phosphatidylinositol 3-kinase/AKT signaling pathway. Journal of Biological Chemistry. 2000;**275**(5):3568-3576

[41] Machens A, Niccoli-Sire P, Hoegel J, Frank-Raue K, van Vroonhoven TJ, Roeher H-D, et al. Early malignant progression of hereditary medullary thyroid cancer. New England Journal of Medicine. 2003;**349**(16):1517-1525

[42] Kouvaraki MA, Shapiro SE, Perrier ND, Cote GJ, Gagel RF, Hoff AO, et al. RET proto-oncogene: a review and update of genotype–phenotype correlations in hereditary medullary thyroid cancer and associated endocrine tumors. Thyroid. 2005;**15**(6):531-544

[43] Figlioli G, Landi S, Romei C, Elisei R, Gemignani F. Medullary thyroid carcinoma (MTC) and RET proto-oncogene: Mutation spectrum in the familial cases and a meta-analysis of studies on the sporadic form. Mutation Research/Reviews in Mutation Research. 2013;**752**(1):36-44

[44] Strosberg JR. Update on the management of unusual neuroendocrine tumors: pheochromocytoma and paraganglioma, medullary thyroid cancer and adrenocortical carcinoma. Seminars in Oncology. 2013;**40**(1): 120-133

[45] Frank-Raue K, Rondot S, Schulze E, Raue F. Change in the spectrum of RET mutations diagnosed between 1994 and 2006. Clinical Laboratory. 2007;**53**(5–6): 273-282

[46] Kloos RT, Eng C, Evans DB, Francis GL, Gagel RF, Gharib H, et al. Medullary thyroid cancer: management guidelines of the American Thyroid Association. Thyroid. 2009;**19**(6): 565-612

[47] Alvandi E, Akrami SM, Chiani M, Hedayati M, Nayer BN, Tehrani MRM, et al. Molecular analysis of the RET proto-oncogene key exons in patients with medullary thyroid carcinoma: A comprehensive study of the Iranian population. Thyroid. 2011;**21**(4):373-382

[48] Sheikholeslami S, Yeganeh MZ, Rad LH, Ghadaksaz HG, Hedayati M. Haplotype Frequency of G691S/S904S in the RET proto-onco-gene in Patients with medullary thyroid carcinoma. Iranian Journal of Public Health. 2014; **43**(2):235

[49] Neocleous V, Skordis N, Portides G, Efstathiou E, Costi C, Ioannou N, et al. RET proto-oncogene mutations are restricted to codon 618 in Cypriot families with multiple endocrine neoplasia 2. Journal of Endocrinological Investigation. 2011;**34**(10):764-769

[50] Zarif Yeganeh M, Sheikholeslami S, Dehbashi Behbahani G, Farashi S, Hedayati M. Skewed mutational spectrum of RET proto-oncogene Exon 10 in Iranian patients with medullary thyroid carcinoma. Tumor Biology. 2015; **36**(7):5225-5231

[51] Hesanmanesh H, Zarif Yeganeh M, Sheikholeslami S, Daneshvar Farhud D, Hedayati M. Germline mutations of RET proto-oncogene exon 2 in iranian population with medullary thyroid carcinoma. Koomesh. 2016;**17**(3): 636-642

[52] Carlomagno F, Vitagliano D, Guida T, Basolo F, Castellone MD, Melillo RM, et al. Efficient inhibition of RET/papillary thyroid carcinoma oncogenic kinases by 4-amino-5-(4-chloro-phenyl)-7-(t-butyl) pyrazolo [3, 4-d] pyrimidine (PP2). The Journal of Clinical Endocrinology and Metabolism. 2003;**88**(4):1897-1902

[53] Cuccuru G, Lanzi C, Cassinelli G, Pratesi G, Tortoreto M, Petrangolini G, et al. Cellular effects and antitumor activity of RET inhibitor RPI-1 on MEN2A-associated medullary thyroid carcinoma. Journal of the National Cancer Institute. 2004;**96**(13): 1006-1014

[54] Strock CJ, Park J-I, Rosen DM, Ruggeri B, Denmeade SR, Ball DW, et al. Activity of irinotecan and the tyrosine kinase inhibitor CEP-751 in medullary thyroid cancer. The Journal of Clinical Endocrinology and Metabolism. 2006; **91**(1):79-84

[55] Lindsey SC, Ganly I, Palmer F, Tuttle RM. Response to initial therapy predicts clinical outcomes in medullary thyroid cancer. Thyroid. 2015;**25**(2): 242-249

[56] Wells SA Jr, Asa SL, Dralle H, Elisei R, Evans DB, Gagel RF, et al. Revised American thyroid association guidelines for the management of medullary thyroid carcinoma: The American thyroid association guidelines task force on medullary thyroid carcinoma. Thyroid. 2015;**25**(6):567-610

[57] Tuttle RM, Haddad RI, Ball DW, Byrd D, Dickson P, Duh Q-Y, et al. Thyroid carcinoma, version 2.2014. Journal of the National Comprehensive Cancer Network. 2014;**12**(12):1671-1680

[58] Frank-Raue K, Buhr H, Dralle H, Klar E, Senninger N, Weber T, et al. Long-term outcome in 46 gene carriers of hereditary medullary thyroid carcinoma after prophylactic thyroidectomy: Impact of individual RET genotype. European Journal of Endocrinology. 2006;**155**(2):229-236

[59] McClellan J, King M-C. Genetic heterogeneity in human disease. Cell. 2010;**141**(2):210-217

[60] Etit D, Faquin WC, Gaz R, Randolph G, DeLellis RA, Pilch BZ. Histopathologic and clinical features of medullary microcarcinoma and C-cell hyperplasia in prophylactic thyroidectomies for medullary carcinoma: A study of 42 cases. Archives of Pathology and Laboratory Medicine. 2008;**132**(11):1767-1773

[61] Quayle FJ, Fialkowski EA, Benveniste R, Moley JF. Pheochromocytoma penetrance varies by RET mutation in MEN 2A. Surgery. 2007;**142**(6):800-805

[62] Learoyd DL, Gosnell J, Elston MS, Saurine TJ, Richardson A, Delbridge LW, et al. Experience of prophylactic thyroidectomy in multiple endocrine neoplasia type 2A kindreds with RET codon 804 mutations. Clinical Endocrinology. 2005;**63**(6):636-641

[63] Marsh DJ, Theodosopoulos G, Martin-Schulte K, Richardson A-L, Philips J, Röher H-D, et al. Genome-wide copy number imbalances identified in familial and sporadic medullary thyroid carcinoma. The Journal of Clinical Endocrinology and Metabolism. 2003; **88**(4):1866-1872

[64] Abdelhakim A, Anne B, Mohamed K, Nadia B, Mohammed T, Taoufiq F, et al. RET genetic screening in patients with medullary thyroid cancer: The Moroccan experience. Journal of Cancer Research and Therapeutics. 2009;**5**(3):198

[65] Benazzouz B, Hafidi A, Benkhira S, Chraibi A, Kadiri A, Hilal L. C634R mutation of the protooncongene RET and molecular diagnosis in multiple endocrine neoplasia type 2 in a large Moroccan family. Bulletin Du Cancer. 2008;**95**(4):457-463

[66] Oliveira MNL, Hemerly JP, Bastos AU, Tamanaha R, Latini FRM, Camacho CP, et al. The RET p. G533C mutation confers predisposition to multiple endocrine neoplasia type 2A in a Brazilian kindred and is able to induce a malignant phenotype in vitro and in vivo. Thyroid. 2011;**21**(9):975-985

[67] Sharma BP, Saranath D. RET gene mutations and polymorphisms in medullary thyroid carcinomas in Indian patients. Journal of Biosciences. 2011; **36**(4):603-611

[68] Siqueira DR, Romitti M, da Rocha AP, Ceolin L, Meotti C, Estivalet A, et al. The RET polymorphic allele S836S is associated with early metastatic disease in patients with hereditary or sporadic medullary thyroid carcinoma. Endocrine-Related Cancer. 2010;**17**(4):953-963

[69] Jindrichova S, Vcelak J, Vlcek P, Neradilova M, Nemec J, Bendlova B. Screening of six risk exons of the RET proto-oncogene in families with medullary thyroid carcinoma in the Czech Republic. Journal of Endocrinology. 2004;**183**(2):257-265

[70] Chatal J-F, Campion L, Kraeber-Bodéré F, Bardet S, Vuillez J-P, Charbonnel B, et al. Survival improvement in patients with medullary thyroid carcinoma who undergo pretargeted anti-carcinoembryonic-

antigen radioimmunotherapy: A collaborative study with the French Endocrine Tumor Group. J Clin Oncol. 2006;**24**(11):1705-1711

[71] Guyétant S, Josselin N, Savagner F, Rohmer V, Michalak S, Saint-André J-P. C-cell hyperplasia and medullary thyroid carcinoma: clinicopathological and genetic correlations in 66 consecutive patients. Modern Pathology. 2003;**16**(8): 756-763

[72] Schuffeneker I, Billaud M, Calender A, Chambe B, Ginet N, Calmettes C, et al. RET proto-oncogene mutations in French MEN 2A and FMTC families. Human Molecular Genetics. 1994;**3**(11):1939-1943

[73] Frank-Raue K, Höppner W, Frilling A, Kotzerke J, Dralle H, Haase R, et al. Mutations of the ret protooncogene in German multiple endocrine neoplasia families: relation between genotype and phenotype. German Medullary Thyroid Carcinoma Study Group. The Journal of Clinical Endocrinology and Metabolism. 1996;**81**(5):1780-1783

[74] Goutas N, Vlachodimitropoulos D, Bouka M, Lazaris AC, Nasioulas G, Gazouli M. BRAF and K-RAS mutation in a Greek papillary and medullary thyroid carcinoma cohort. Anticancer Research. 2008;**28**(1A):305-308

[75] Kaldrymides P, Mytakidis N, Anagnostopoulos T, Vassiliou M, Tertipi A, Zahariou M, et al. A rare RET gene exon 8 mutation is found in two Greek kindreds with familial medullary thyroid carcinoma: Implications for screening. Clinical Endocrinology. 2006; **64**(5):561-566

[76] Sarika HL, Papathoma A, Garofalaki M, Vasileiou V, Vlassopoulou B, Anastasiou E, et al. High prevalence of exon 8 G 533 C mutation in apparently sporadic medullary thyroid carcinoma in G reece. Clinical Endocrinology. 2012;**77**(6):857-862

[77] Ghazi AA, Bagheri M, Tabibi A, Sarvghadi F, Abdi H, Hedayati M, et al. Multiple endocrine neoplasia type 2A in an Iranian family: clinical and genetic studies. Archives of Iranian Medicine. 2014;**17**(5):0

[78] Hedayati M, Nabipour I, Rezaei-Ghaleh N, Azizi F. Germline RET mutations in exons 10 and 11: an Iranian survey of 57 medullary thyroid carcinoma cases. Medical Journal of Malaysia. 2006;**61**(5):564

[79] Majidi M, Haghpanah V, Hedayati M, Khashayar P, Mohajeri-Tehrani MR, Larijani B. A family presenting with multiple endocrine neoplasia type 2B: A case report. Journal of Medical Case Reports. 2011;**5**(1):1-3

[80] Romei C, Mariotti S, Fugazzola L, Taccaliti A, Pacini F, Opocher G, et al. Multiple endocrine neoplasia type 2 syndromes (MEN 2): results from the Ita MEN network analysis on the prevalence of different genotypes and phenotypes. European Journal of Endocrinology. 2010;**163**(2):301-308

[81] Shifrin AL, Ogilvie JB, Stang MT, Fay AM, Kuo Y-H, Matulewicz T, et al. Single nucleotide polymorphisms act as modifiers and correlate with the development of medullary and simultaneous medullary/papillary thyroid carcinomas in 2 large, non-related families with the RET V804M proto-oncogene mutation. Surgery. 2010;**148**(6):1274-1281

[82] Kameyama K, Okinaga H, Takami H. RET oncogene mutations in 75 cases of familial medullary thyroid carcinoma in Japan. Biomedicine and Pharmacotherapy. 2004;**58**(6–7): 345-347

[83] González-Yebra B, Medrano ME, Mantilla A, Palma V, Colin C, Hernández DM, et al. Penetrance of inherited medullary thyroid carcinoma and genotype-phenotype correlation in a large multiple endocrine neoplasia type 2A family with C634Y RET mutatiom. Endocrine Pathology. 2003;**14**(1):71-80

[84] Jae Chung Y, Kim H-H, Kim H-J, Min Y-K, Lee M-S, Lee M-K, et al. RET proto-oncogene mutations are restricted to codon 634 and 618 in Korean families with multiple endocrine neoplasia 2A. Thyroid. 2004;**14**(10):813-818

[85] Jung J, Uchino S, Lee Y, Park H. A Korean family of familial medullary thyroid cancer with Cys618Ser RET germline mutation. Journal of Korean Medical Science. 2010;**25**(2):226-229

[86] Bugalho MJ, Domingues R, Santos JR, Catarino AL, Sobrinho L. Mutation analysis of the RET proto-oncogene and early thyroidectomy: Results of a Portuguese cancer centre. Surgery. 2007;**141**(1):90-95

[87] Prazeres HJ, Rodrigues F, Figueiredo P, Naidenov P, Soares P, Bugalho MJ, et al. Occurrence of the Cys611Tyr mutation and a novel Arg 886Trp substitution in the RET proto-oncogene in multiple endocrine neoplasia type 2 families and sporadic medullary thyroid carcinoma cases originating from the central region of Portugal. Clinical Endocrinology. 2006; **64**(6):659-666

[88] Silva AL, Carmo F, Moura MM, Domingues R, Espadinha C, Leite V, et al. Identification and characterization of two novel germline RET variants associated with medullary thyroid carcinoma. Endocrine. 2015;**49**(2):366-372

[89] Moore SW, Zaahl MG. Multiple endocrine neoplasia syndromes, children, Hirschsprung's disease and RET. Pediatric Surgery International. 2008;**24**(5):521-530

[90] Moore SW, Zaahl MG. Chasing the ubiquitous RET proto-oncogene in South African MEN2 families-implications for the surgeon: oncology. South African Journal of Surgery. 2010;**48**(4):127-131

[91] Moore SW, Appfelstaedt J, Zaahl MG. Familial medullary carcinoma prevention, risk evaluation, and RET in children of families with MEN2. Journal of Pediatric Surgery. 2007;**42**(2):326-332

[92] Belli S, Storani ME, Dourisboure RJ, Podestá EJ, Solano AR. Study of RET protooncogene in multiple endocrine neoplasm 2A and in familial medullary thyroid carcinoma. Clinical pathological findings in asymptomatic carriers. Medicina. 2003;**63**(1):41-45

[93] Milos IN, Frank-Raue K, Wohllk N, Maia AL, Pusiol E, Patocs A, et al. Age-related neoplastic risk profiles and penetrance estimations in multiple endocrine neoplasia type 2A caused by germ line RET Cys634Trp (TGC> TGG) mutation. Endocrine-Related Cancer. 2008;**15**(4):1035-1041

[94] Nelson Wohllk G, Youlton R, Cote GJ, Gagel RF. Germline mutations of the ret proto-oncogen in Chilean patients with hereditary and sporadic medullary thyroid carcinoma. Rev. Méd. Chile. 2001;**129**(7)

[95] Sobrino PS, Fernández CP, Gil PG, Gil BM, Pedrosa AP, Carballeira RP, et al. Phenotype of the C634Y mutation in the RET proto-oncogene in MEN2A: Report of a family. Endocrinología y Nutrición (English Edition). 2011;**58**(5): 229-235

Chapter 3

Genomics Underlying Familial Thyroid Carcinoma in Dogs

Yun Yu and Richard R.P.A. Crooijmans

Abstract

Thyroid cancer is the most common endocrine neoplasm occurring in dogs. We reported familial thyroid follicular cell carcinomas (FCCs) in 54 Dutch German longhaired pointer (GLP) dogs. We investigated the genetics of the FCC in these dogs, including the germline risk mutations and somatic driver mutations. We identified the germline risk factor locating in the *TPO* gene for these hereditary FCCs through a combination of genome-wide association study (GWAS) and homozygosity mapping analyses using SNP array genotype data and whole-genome sequencing data. We further investigated the somatic mutation landscape of these FCCs using high-depth whole-genome sequencing technology of the tumors. A recurrent missense mutation in the *GNAS* gene was identified as a very promising driver mutation. We validated this somatic mutation using Sanger sequencing and revealed a prevalence of 62.5% among thyroid tumors identified in the Dutch GLPs. In addition, we can also review the findings in genetics of other canine thyroid tumors in recent years.

Keywords: thyroid carcinoma, dog, animal, germline risk factor, somatic mutation

1. Introduction

Dogs have a pair of thyroid glands that are located on each side of windpipe in the neck. Dogs, like humans, develop thyroid cancers in these glands. Thyroid cancer is the most common endocrine neoplasm, accounting for 1%–4% of all canine neoplasms [1]. Thyroid neoplasms can be classified as adenomas or carcinomas. Adenoma is a benign neoplasm, and carcinoma is malignant. Carcinomas are distinguished from adenomas by capsular and/or vascular invasion. Approximately 60%–90% of canine thyroid neoplasms are carcinomas [1]. The thyroid cancer in dogs can be unilateral or bilateral, which account for 67%–75% and 25%–35%, respectively [2]. The typical clinical sign of a thyroid tumor in dogs is the palpable mass in the neck. Other clinical complaints related to thyroid carcinoma include intermittent cough, alopecia, polyuria, polydipsia, weight loss [3].

A canine thyroid tumor can originate from either follicular cells or C-cells (parafollicular cells) in thyroid gland. Thyroid tumors in dogs consist of mainly eight histological subtypes according to a classification of World Health Organization [4], and they are highly similar to corresponding types in humans in histological growth pattern. There are seven subtypes of thyroid tumor originating from follicular cells, including follicular thyroid carcinoma (FTC), papillary thyroid carcinoma (PTC), compact

IntechOpen

thyroid carcinoma (CTC), follicular-compact thyroid carcinoma (FCTC), poorly differentiated thyroid carcinoma, undifferentiated (anaplastic) thyroid carcinoma, and carcinosarcoma. The thyroid cancer originating from C-cells is called medullary thyroid carcinoma (MTC). Most of canine thyroid tumor originates from follicular cells, accounting for 64%–71%, which is also called non-medullary thyroid carcinoma (NMTC). Thyroglobulin is a protein made by the follicular cells of the thyroid gland, and calcitonin is made by C-cells [5, 6]. Thyroglobulin and calcitonin immunohistochemistry experiments are useful to differentiate thyroid cancer originating from follicular cells or C-cells. Thyroid carcinoma originating from follicular cells exhibits positive immunolabeling for thyroglobulin, and MTC exhibits strong immunoreactivity for calcitonin [1].

Thyroid neoplasms in dogs are usually non-functional. Clinical or biochemical evidence of hyperthyroidism can be observed in less than 25% of affected dogs. Meanwhile, hypothyroidism is also possible because of destruction of normal thyroid tissue, suppression of thyroid-stimulating hormone (TSH) secretion, and subsequent atrophy of normal thyroid tissue [2].

Metastasis is common in canine thyroid carcinoma. Approximately one out of three dog patients have metastasis by the time of diagnosis [1, 7], and 65%–90% of untreated dogs are diagnosed with regional or distant metastasis at necropsy [2]. The lung and regional lymph nodes are the most common organs where canine thyroid carcinoma metastasizes to. Metastasis to other organs is occasionally seen, such as the adrenal glands, liver, heart, brain, kidneys, and bone [1]. In dogs, risk of thyroid tumor increases with age. The average age at diagnosis is between 9 and 10 years. Dogs at age > 10 years have a significantly higher risk of thyroid cancer than younger dogs [1, 8].

Canine thyroid tumors show also some differences if compared with humans. For instance, in humans, females have approximately 2–3 times higher risk for non-medullary thyroid cancer than males [9]. While, in dogs, most studies reported equal incidence of thyroid carcinoma in both sexes [3, 8]. The mechanism underlying the sex bias in incidence of thyroid cancer in humans is still unclear. Another difference is that the most prevalent subtype of thyroid cancer is different between humans and dogs. In humans, PTC is the most frequently diagnosed thyroid cancer, accounting for approximately 85%–90% [10]. However, in dogs, PTC is relatively rare, and FTC is the most common type of thyroid carcinoma [1].

2. A familial canine thyroid carcinoma

Reports of hereditary thyroid carcinoma in dogs are limited. One report presented a hereditary canine MTC with a potential dominant inheritance of autosomal or X-linked inheritance in a family of a mixed dog breed with Alaskan malamute as a major influence [11]. We reported a hereditary thyroid follicular cell carcinoma in a large number of Dutch German longhaired pointer (GLP) dogs [3]. Over the past ~20 years, thyroid tumor was identified in 84 Dutch GLPs. Among those affected GLPs, 54 had histologically diagnosed thyroid follicular cell carcinomas (FCCs), 29 were suspected cases solely based on clinical diagnosis (such as palpable mass in the neck), and 1 had thyroid adenoma. The identified histology subtypes of the FCC include FTC, CTC, FCTC, PTC, and carcinosarcoma. The same as findings in other studies about canine thyroid tumor [1], FTC is the most common among all these subtypes, accounting for 46%. Meanwhile, no sex predisposition was observed in those affected GLPs. Canine FTC

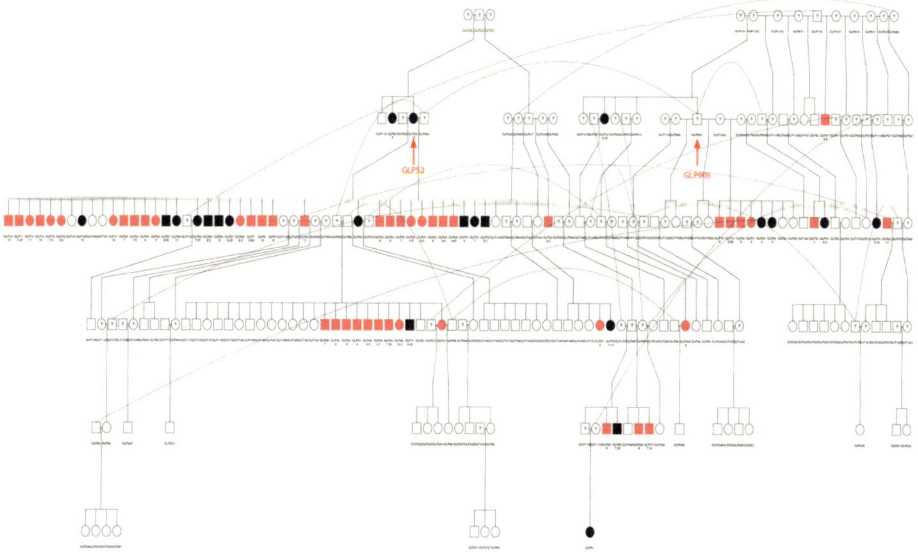

Figure 1.
Pedigree of dogs related to two dogs (pointed by red arrows) that were intensively used in breeding [3]. Forty-five histopathologically confirmed affected dogs are closely related to these two dogs. Circles represent females, and squares represent males. Dot line shows identical dogs. Affected dogs with histological diagnosis are highlighted in red, and suspected affected dogs (without histopathology diagnosis) are in black, whereas unaffected dogs remain white. A question mark represents the dogs with unknown status.

incidence increases with age where approximately 57% of cases were diagnosed at ages between 10 and 15 years. However, FCCs in these GLPs were diagnosed earlier where 76% of cases were diagnosed before 10 years of age.

These affected GLPs are very closely related in terms of genetic relationship, where many of them are first-degree relatives, suggesting that these FCCs belong to a familial form of thyroid carcinoma (**Figure 1**). In humans, a hereditary thyroid cancer is diagnosed when there are two or more first-degree relatives affected [12]. In dogs, according to authors' knowledge, there is no definition of a hereditary thyroid cancer yet. The definition of hereditary thyroid carcinoma in humans can be borrowed. A striking high incidence of the FCC in offspring of two GLPs was seen (**Figure 1**). Most of identified affected dogs are related to these two GLPs in pedigree. In the past, in dog breeding, some prominent dogs were used intensively including breeding with relatives, which resulted in the introduction of genetic defects and spread unwanted diseases in the population. The familial FCC here is a good example.

3. Germline risk factor of the familial FCC

Cancer is a disease caused by one or multiple mutation(s) in the genome of cells. A familial cancer has one or multiple germline causal mutations that are inherited from parents of the individual. Identification of germline causal variants has important value for both cancer prevention factors of human thyroid cancer. GWAS is a statistical method to identify genomic regions that are associated with targeted traits/disease taking advantage of linkage disequilibrium between genomic variants.

Linkage disequilibrium is the non-random association of alleles at different genomic loci in a given population. It makes it possible to identify the genomic region associated with the investigated trait/disease even when the causal loci are not genotyped. After a GWAS analysis, fine-mapping can be performed to identify the causal variants in the targeted genomic region. Whole-genome sequencing data are usually used in fine-mapping, which can identify all the variants when compared with the reference genome. In order to confirm the causal variants and underlying molecular mechanism, further *in vitro* or *in vivo* experiments are needed., diagnosis, and novel drug development. Next-generation sequencing technologies make it easy to obtain whole-genome sequencing data of an individual. However, identification of germline causal mutations for a disease/cancer is still challenging. In the past decade, many genome-wide association studies (GWASs) have been performed to identify germline risk.

Identification of germline risk factor of a hereditary form of thyroid cancer is still challenging. In humans, only approximately 5% of a form of familial non-medullary thyroid cancers have well-documented germline risk factors [13]. We performed a series of analyses based on a combination of SNP array genotype data and whole-genome sequencing data to identify the germline risk mutation that confers a higher risk for thyroid carcinoma in Dutch GLPs [14]. We combined a GWAS analysis and a homozygosity mapping to identify the genomic region that is associated with the FCC. This combined strategy was used because clear population stratification was observed between the genotyped affected and unaffected dogs. In the GWAS analysis, to correct over false-positive discoveries, genomic relationship matrix estimated based on genotype data was incorporated as a random effect. Homozygosity mapping was also used because the FCC in these dogs has very likely an autosomal recessive inheritance pattern according to pedigree. Homozygosity mapping used in that study is based on runs of homozygosity (ROH)-based approach, which is a powerful method to identify genomic region that is associated with a recessive disease. A common genomic region was identified by both the GWAS and homozygosity mapping analyses. Next, we performed fine-mapping using WGS data of 11 affected and 11 unaffected GLPs to identify the germline mutations that are in the targeted region. A series of stringent filtering was performed on the variants identified in the targeted

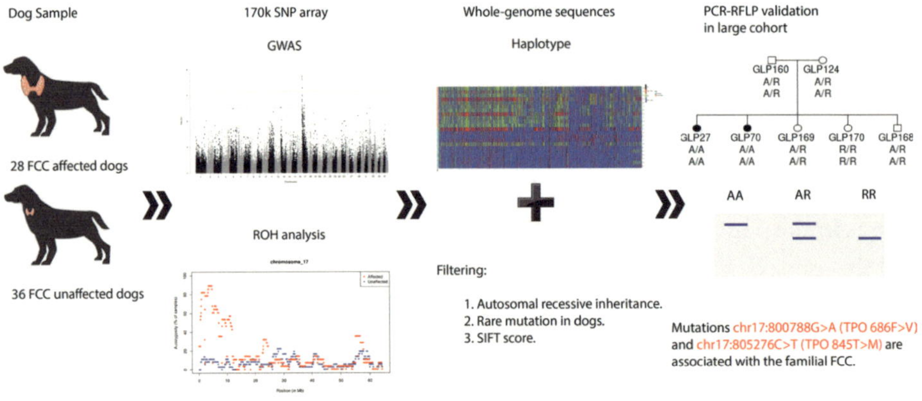

Figure 2.
Graphic abstract of identification of the germline risk mutations in the familial FCC [14]. 170K SNP array genotype data were obtained from 36 healthy German longhaired pointer (GLP) dogs and 28 GLPs affected by the familial thyroid follicular cell carcinoma. The genotype data were used in the genome-wide association analysis and homozygosity mapping to identify genomic region associated with the familial thyroid follicular cell carcinoma.

genomic region based on WGS data: 1) must be deleterious predicted by pathogenicity prediction tools; 2) must fit an autosomal recessive inheritance pattern; 3) must be rare in general dogs; 4) must be conserved across species. At the end, we identified two deleterious mutations, chr17:800788G>A (p.686F>V) and chr17:805276C>T (p.845T>M), in the *TPO* gene. We further genotyped these two variants in 186 GLPs (59 affected and 127 unaffected) using PCR-RFLP experiment and revealed 16.94 and 16.64 of the relative risk of homozygous recessive genotypes compared with homozygous genotypes for the reference allele (**Figure 2**).

The genetic cause of general canine thyroid cancer is still poorly studied. There is no study that investigated the genetic causes of canine thyroid cancer at a genome-wide scale, except for our study. Genetic causes of canine thyroid cancer need to be revealed since thyroid tumor is the most frequent endocrine neoplasm in dogs.

4. Somatic mutations in canine thyroid cancer

Most of thyroid carcinomas in dogs are sporadic, the same as it is in humans. Sporadic cancers are caused by somatic mutations that occur in somatic cells, which are different from germline causal mutations in hereditary cancers. These somatic mutations are not inherited from parents of the individual, but are acquired by random DNA replication error during cell divisions that occurred by chance or due to exogenous or endogenous carcinogens that can increase the risk for the cancer. These exogenous carcinogens include smoking and X-ray. Endogenous carcinogen includes reactive oxygen species produced during metabolism [15]. When these mutations occur in proto-oncogene or tumor-suppressor gene, then a cancerous cell may arise.

Identification of somatic mutation at a genome-wide scale becomes possible with the development of next-generation sequencing technologies. The Cancer Genome Atlas (TCGA) and International Cancer Genome Consortium (ICGC) projects have profiled tens of thousands of human cancers of different types and origins [16, 17]. Normally, whole-genome or whole-exome sequences of tumor tissue and matched normal tissue (blood or healthy tissue adjacent to tumor tissue) are generated and compared to identify those somatic mutations that are unique to tumor cells. Among somatic mutations, according to their role in tumorigenesis, driver and passenger mutations are defined. Driver mutations are somatic mutations that are important to the tumor initiation and growth, and passenger mutations are those neutral mutations that do not contribute to tumorigenesis. Identification of driver mutation is one of the major tasks in oncogenic research. Identification of driver mutations sheds light on molecular mechanisms underlying tumor initiation and development. Those driver mutations have potential value to be used to develop targeted treatment to kill cancerous cells.

Somatic mutations of human thyroid carcinoma have been extensively investigated at a genome-wide scale. Somatic mutations of canine thyroid carcinoma are still poorly studied. A somatic mutation in *P53* gene has been identified in canine FTC [18]. We profiled the somatic mutations of the hereditary FCC identified in Dutch GLPs at a genome-wide scale [19]. As far as we know, there was no genome-wide profile of somatic mutations in canine thyroid carcinoma before our study. In our study, a missense somatic mutation in the *GNAS* gene, p.A204D, stands up where it was identified in four of seven FCC samples that were whole-genome sequenced and validated in 20 out of the 32 affected dogs' thyroid tumor samples [19]. This high prevalence of the somatic mutation is a strong evidence of the driver role of this mutation in these canine thyroid carcinomas.

The *GNAS* gene encodes the alpha-subunit of stimulatory G-protein (Gαs) that can activate adenylyl cyclase downstream of G-protein-coupled receptors (GPCRs). Activated adenylyl cyclase increases cellular cyclic adenosine monophosphate (cAMP). cAMP is an important second messenger that can upregulate many downstream molecular signaling cascades, including pathways involved in cell proliferation, such as the PKA signaling pathway [20].

The *GNAS* gene is a known proto-oncogene. Somatic mutations in the *GNAS* gene have been identified in many different types of tumors in humans. It is known that activating mutations in the *GNAS* gene can result in increased cell division in humans. The most common activating mutations in the *GNAS* identified in human tumors are p.R201C/H/S and p.Q227R/L [21]. According to an investigation in 274,694 human tumors, appendiceal adenocarcinoma has highest frequency of *GNAS* activating mutation (35.9%). Ovarian carcinosarcoma, rectum adenocarcinoma, gastroesophageal junction adenocarcinoma, stomach adenocarcinoma diffuse type, small intestine adenocarcinoma, stomach adenocarcinoma, esophagus adenocarcinoma, breast carcinoma, colon adenocarcinoma, breast invasive ductal carcinoma, and duodenal adenocarcinoma have prevalence of *GNAS* somatic mutation in the range between 5% and 7% [21]. However, prevalence of somatic mutation in the *GNAS* gene in human thyroid cancer seems to be low where only 13 of 1,837 human thyroid neoplasms capture *GNAS* somatic mutations. Likewise, somatic mutations in the *GNAS* gene were identified in only two out of 496 PTC samples that were included in the TCGA project [22].

Besides our genome-wide study, Campos et al. investigated somatic mutation landscape of 43 canine FCCs and 16 canine MTCs by targeted sequencing of some driver genes identified in human thyroid carcinoma [23]. Those genes include *HRAS*, *KRAS*, *PIK3CA*, *BRAF*, *RET*, and *PTEN* genes. However, they only identified two missense mutations in the *KRAS* gene that are homologous to mutations identified in human thyroid carcinoma. No somatic mutation in other genes under investigation was identified. This seems to suggest that canine thyroid carcinoma uses different driver mutations compared with human thyroid carcinoma. In our study, *GNAS* p.A204D somatic mutation was observed in FCC neoplasms of 62.5% of affected GLPs. However, in human PTCs, *GNAS* somatic mutation is rarely observed. This suggests the potential difference in driver events of thyroid carcinoma between humans and GLPs. We suggest that the prevalence of the *GNAS* somatic mutation in more canine thyroid tumors should be investigated because it might be a major driver mutation of canine thyroid tumor according to our study. Meanwhile, we also suggest investigating driver mutations in sporadic canine thyroid carcinomas at a genome-wide scale to elucidate the molecular mechanisms underlying canine sporadic thyroid tumor initiation and development and to investigate the potential value of dogs with sporadic thyroid carcinoma to be used as disease models.

5. Pathways involved in thyroid carcinoma in dogs

In humans, molecular signaling pathways that are involved in thyroid carcinoma are extensively investigated. The most dominant molecular signaling pathways are the mitogen-activated protein kinase (MAPK) and phosphatidylinositol-3 kinase (PI3K)/Akt pathways [24]. Activation of these pathways as a result of activating mutations in proto-oncogenes (such as *BRAF* and *RAS* genes) involved in the pathway leads to cancerous cells. In dogs, PI3K/AKT pathway is also involved in the pathogenesis of thyroid carcinoma with the evidence of increased expression of several genes associated with the pathway [23]. However, the involvement of MAPK pathway in canine thyroid carcinoma development needs to be investigated. Besides the evidence of increased expression of genes, to confirm the role of these pathways in the canine thyroid carcinoma development, somatic mutations in those genes should also be further investigated.

6. Inbreeding and disease incidence

Inbreeding is the production of offspring from mating or breeding of individuals or organisms that are closely related [25]. It can be technically defined as mating of a pair of animals with relationship that is closer than the average level within the breed or population studied. In domesticated animals, inbreeding can decrease the performance of animals, such as decrease in milk yield, which is termed as inbreeding depression. The genetic basis of inbreeding depression is that increased homozygosity with inbreeding increases the frequency of unfavorable genotypes within the population [25]. Inbreeding can increase the incidence of inherited diseases in the population, especially those with a recessive inheritance pattern. In our studies, we estimated inbreeding coefficients using either pedigree or genome-wide genotype data. We observed significantly higher inbreeding levels in affected GLPs (average pedigree-based inbreeding: 0.23, average genotype-based inbreeding: 0.51) in comparison to those unaffected GLPs (average pedigree-based inbreeding: 0.14, average genotype-based inbreeding: 0.48). This suggests the importance of inbreeding control in preventing inherited diseases, including cancer, in pedigree dog breeding.

7. The usage of identified germline and somatic mutations

Identification of germline risk mutations can be valuable for cancer prevention. For hereditary cancer with a simple inheritance pattern, the identified germline risk mutation can be used to identify those individuals that have a higher risk for the cancer through a genetic test. Those animals then can be removed from the breeding program to eradicate the inherited cancer from the population. Without a genetic test, it is hard to completely remove a disease with an autosomal recessive inheritance pattern from the population because of difficulty in identifying those heterozygous animals. For a cancer with a complex inheritance pattern, a polygenic risk score can be calculated based on all identified germline risk mutations to predict the risk of the cancer development for an individual. For those people with a high risk score for certain disease, early prevention, such as healthy dietaries and life styles, can be taken to diminish the risk. Frequent examination can also be arranged to detect the disease earlier and cure easier.

We developed a genetic test based on one of the germline risk mutation (chr17:800788G>A) in the *TPO* gene to identify GLPs that have a higher risk for the FCC. This genetic test is now commercially available for GLP breeders and owners after testing 142 GLPs at the Animal Breeding and Genomics laboratory. To date, this genetic test has been performed on more than 150 GLPs from a few countries. The frequency of germline risk allele is 25.4% in those tested GLPs. This frequency is rather high and indicates that the risk allele is hard to be completely eradicated from the population by conventional breeding strategy. The genetic test can be especially valuable for GLP breeders to breed healthy dogs. It enables breeders to find those dogs at a high risk for the FCC before any signs of the disease and then those dogs can be excluded from the breeding program.

8. Germline and somatic mutation interaction

TPO gene encodes an enzyme, thyroid peroxidase, which plays an important role in production of thyroid hormones. There are seven key steps in the thyroid hormone synthesis: 1) iodine uptake into thyroid follicular cells by the sodium/iodide symporter (NIS); 2) synthesis of two key proteins, thyroid peroxidase (TPO) and thyroglobulin (TG), and secretion of TG into the follicular lumen; 3) iodide transport into the follicular lumen; 4) iodide oxidation to form iodine by TPO; 5) iodination of TG tyrosine residues to generate monoiodotyrosine (MIT) and diiodotyrosine (DIT) by TPO; 6) coupling of iodotyrosines to form thyroxine (T4) and triiodothyronine (T3) by TPO; 7) endocytosis of TG-thyroid hormone complex and T3 and T4 cleaved from it by proteases in the lysosomes [26, 27]. TPO is involved in steps 4, 5, and 6. Meanwhile, hydrogen peroxide (H_2O_2) is needed in those reactions catalyzed by the TPO. We suspect that germline mutations identified in the *TPO* gene may impair the activity of the TPO enzyme and result in less consumption of H_2O_2, therefore increased level of H_2O_2. This assumption needs to be validated in future using, for instance, cell experiments. However, hydrogen peroxide is a type of reactive oxygen species that can induce DNA damages. Elevated H_2O_2 probably induces many somatic mutations occurring in the thyroid follicular cells and finally a cancerous cell form when a driver mutation occurs. In those familial FCCs, one of driver mutations is the recurrent somatic mutation identified in the *GNAS* gene.

9. Medullary thyroid cancer in dogs

Regarding MTC, both spontaneous and hereditary forms have been reported in dogs [7, 11, 28, 29]. Up to 20%–30% of human hereditary MTC is caused by activating mutations in the *RET* proto-oncogene [30]. In the hereditary MTCs that were studied by Lee et al., the authors sequenced the *RET* gene but identified no mutation in that gene [11]. The germline genetic causes of canine MTC including the somatic driver mutations are still not clear. Canine familial MTC is similar to human familial MTC in clinical symptoms and morphology of histology, suggesting their value to be used as a disease model. However, unraveling the genetic basis of canine MTC is needed for that purpose.

10. Thyroid cancer in other species

Besides the occurrence in dogs, thyroid tumor has also been reported in many other species, such as guinea pig [31], cat [32], horse [33], cattle [34, 35], barred owl [36], rat [37], and ferret [38, 39]. Thyroid hyperplasia was seen in fish over one hundred years ago, and thyroid neoplasms were also reported in fish [40]. Thyroid carcinoma has been induced in mice using transgenic technology for the study of pathogenesis [41]. Genetic causes of thyroid carcinoma in these species (except for mice) are generally not known. Mapping of the genetic causes of thyroid carcinoma in these species is needed to elucidate the molecular mechanism of tumorigenesis. However, it is challenging due to the difficulty in identifying sufficient amount of cases for causal mutation mapping in those species.

11. Dogs as cancer models

An animal model is an indispensable model to investigate the pathogenesis, molecular mechanisms of tumor initiation and development and to test novel treatments. Scientists have increasing interest in dog disease models in recent years. Dogs may have many advantages to be used as disease models compared with the most popular model species such as mouse and rat [42]. Dogs are the most popular companion animals globally and are the second in medical surveillance and preventative health care after humans [42]. Dogs are more similar to humans such as in genetics, immune systems, body size. Meanwhile, pet dogs share living environment with their owners, thus receiving similar environment factors. There is, for example, a gap between mouse model and chimpanzee models in clinical trials. There is no doubt that mice contribute a lot to novel drug development. However, it is also true that many drugs work during trials on mice but fail in human clinical trials because of difference in physiology between these two species.

Breed dogs have in general low genetic diversity due to two bottleneck events in history: one is domestication from grey wolf around 15,000 years ago, and another one is strong artificial selection in order to fix certain traits of breeds during the breed formation in the past ~200 years [43]. This low genetic diversity results in many genetic diseases/disorders, such as osteosarcoma in Rottweiler, elbow dysplasia in Labrador Retriever, and medial patellar luxation in Chihuahua [44, 45]. According to a study of Farrell et al., there are 396 hereditary disorders identified in 215 officially recognized dog breeds in the United Kingdom [46]. Many of these disorders also occur in humans, which makes those dogs potentially valuable disease models to investigate the pathogenesis of those disorders. Low genetic diversity within each dog breed makes mapping of causal variants of those diseases easier in dogs than that in humans. Much smaller number of SNPs are needed to identify the genomic region that is associated with an inherited disease in dogs in comparison to humans because of the low genetic diversity and large haplotype blocks [42]. This facilitates unraveling the genetic basis of inherited disease.

In rodents, thyroid carcinoma usually has a follicular architecture but does not have the morphological or cytological characteristics used in the diagnosis of papillary carcinomas in humans [37]. Canine thyroid carcinoma is more similar to human thyroid carcinoma in morphology of histology in comparison to thyroid carcinoma in rodents. GLPs with familial FCCs can be a valuable disease model to elucidate the molecular mechanism underlying tumor initiation and development with driver mutations in the *GNAS* gene.

12. Conclusion

We summarized our research regarding a familial thyroid follicular cell carcinoma in Dutch German longhaired pointer dogs. We identified two deleterious mutations in the *TPO* gene that confer great relative risk in homozygous status. A genetic test was developed and made commercially available for breeders and owners of GLPs. We expect to greatly diminish the incidence of the familial FCC in GLPs by using this genetic test and will help to eradicate the familial FCC from the GLP population. Furthermore, we identified a recurrent somatic mutation, the *GNAS* p.A204D, in the familial FCCs with a prevalence of 62.5%. Identification of this somatic mutation implicates the role of GPCR-mediated molecular signaling pathways in the FCC initiation and development. With a high prevalence of the *GNAS* p.A204D somatic mutation, those affected dogs might serve as a good disease model to understand the pathogenesis of tumors associated with *GNAS* somatic mutations and to test novel treatments that targets on tumors with *GNAS* somatic mutations.

Conflict of interest

The authors declare no conflict of interest.

Author details

Yun Yu and Richard R.P.A. Crooijmans*
Animal Breeding and Genomics, Wageningen University, Wageningen, The Netherlands

*Address all correspondence to: richard.crooijmans@wur.nl

References

[1] Hassan BB, Altstadt LA, Dirksen WP, Elshafae SM, Rosol TJ. Canine thyroid cancer: Molecular characterization and cell line growth in nude mice. Veterinary Pathology. 2020;**57**(2):227-240

[2] Liptak JM. Canine thyroid carcinoma. Clinical Techniques in Small Animal Practice. 2007;**22**(2):75-81

[3] Yu Y, Krupa A, Keesler RI, Grinwis GCM, de Ruijsscher M, de Vos J, et al. Familial follicular cell thyroid carcinomas in a large number of Dutch German longhaired pointers. Veterinary and Comparative Oncology. 2022;**20**(1):227-234

[4] Kiupel M, Capen C, Miller M, Smedley R. Histological Classification of Tumors of the Endocrine System of Domestic Animals. Armed Forces Inst. of Pathology; 2008

[5] Peiris AN, Medlock D, Gavin M. Thyroglobulin for monitoring for thyroid cancer recurrence. JAMA. 2019;**321**(12):1228

[6] Garrett JE, Tamir H, Kifor O, Simin RT, Rogers KV, Mithal A, et al. Calcitonin-secreting cells of the thyroid express an extracellular calcium receptor gene. Endocrinology. 1995;**136**(11):5202-5211

[7] Campos M, Ducatelle R, Kooistra HS, Rutteman G, Duchateau L, Polis I, et al. Immunohistochemical Expression of Potential Therapeutic Targets in Canine Thyroid Carcinoma. Journal of Veterinary Internal Medicine. 2014;**28**(2):564-570

[8] Wucherer KL, Wilke V. Thyroid cancer in dogs: An update based on 638 cases (1995-2005). Journal of the American Animal Hospital Association. 2010;**46**(4):249-254

[9] Patel S, Pappoppula L, Guddati AK, Annamaraju P. Analysis of race and gender disparities in incidence-based mortality in patients diagnosed with thyroid cancer from 2000 to 2016. International Journal of General Medicine. 2020;**13**:1589-1594

[10] Pusztaszeri M, Auger M. Update on the cytologic features of papillary thyroid carcinoma variants. Diagnostic Cytopathology. 2017;**45**(8):714-730

[11] Lee J-J, Larsson C, Lui W-O, Höög A, Von Euler H. A dog pedigree with familial medullary thyroid cancer. International Journal of Oncology. 2006;**29**(5):1173-1182

[12] Nosé V. Familial thyroid cancer: A review. Modern Pathology. 2011;**24**:S19

[13] Guilmette J, Nosé V. Hereditary and familial thyroid tumours. Histopathology. 2018;**72**(1):70-81

[14] Yu Y, Bovenhuis H, Wu Z, Laport K, Groenen MAM, Crooijmans RPMA. Deleterious mutations in the TPO gene associated with familial thyroid follicular cell carcinoma in dutch german longhaired pointers. Genes. 2021;**12**(7):997

[15] Martincorena I, Campbell PJ. Somatic mutation in cancer and normal cells. Science. 2015;**349**(6255):1483-1489

[16] Weinstein JN, Collisson EA, Mills GB, Shaw KR, Ozenberger BA, Ellrott K, et al. The cancer genome Atlas Pan-cancer analysis project. Nature Genetics. 2013;**45**(10):1113-1120

[17] Hudson TJ, Anderson W, Artez A, Barker AD, Bell C, Bernabé RR, et al. International network of cancer genome projects. Nature. 2010;**464**(7291):993-998

[18] Devilee P, Van Leeuwen IS, Voesten A, Rutteman GR, Vos JH, Cornelisse CJ. The canine p53 gene is subject to somatic mutations in thypoid carcinoma. Anticancer Research. 1994;**14**(5a):2039-2046

[19] Yu Y, Manders F, Grinwis GCM, Groenen MAM, Crooijmans RPMA. A recurrent somatic missense mutation in GNAS gene identified in familial thyroid follicular cell carcinomas in German longhaired pointer dogs. BMC Genomics. 2022;**23**(1):669

[20] Turan S, Bastepe M. GNAS spectrum of disorders. Current Osteoporosis Reports. 2015;**13**(3):146-158

[21] Tirosh A, Jin DX, De Marco L, Laitman Y, Friedman E. Activating genomic alterations in the Gs alpha gene (GNAS) in 274 694 tumors. Genes, Chromosomes & Cancer. 2020;**59**(9):503-516

[22] Agrawal N, Akbani R, Aksoy BA, Ally A, Arachchi H, Asa Sylvia L, et al. Integrated genomic characterization of papillary thyroid carcinoma. Cell. 2014;**159**(3):676-690

[23] Campos M, Kool MMJ, Daminet S, Ducatelle R, Rutteman G, Kooistra HS, et al. Upregulation of the PI3K/Akt pathway in the tumorigenesis of canine thyroid carcinoma. Journal of Veterinary Internal Medicine. 2014;**28**(6):1814-1823

[24] Zaballos MA, Santisteban P. Key signaling pathways in thyroid cancer. The Journal of Endocrinology. 2017;**235**(2):R43-R61

[25] Doekes HP, Veerkamp RF, Bijma P, de Jong G, Hiemstra SJ, Windig JJ. Inbreeding depression due to recent and ancient inbreeding in Dutch Holstein–Friesian dairy cattle. Genetics, Selection, Evolution. 2019;**51**(1):54

[26] Rousset B, Dupuy C, Miot F, Dumont J. Chapter 2 Thyroid hormone synthesis and secretion. In: Feingold KR, Anawalt B, Boyce A, Chrousos G, de Herder WW, Dhatariya K, et al., editors. Endotext. South Dartmouth (MA): MDText.com, Inc, 2000

[27] Koibuchi N. Molecular mechanisms of thyroid hormone synthesis and secretion. Nihon Rinsho. 2012;**70**(11):1844-1848

[28] Arias ES, Castillo V, Trigo R, Aristarain MC. Multiple endocrine neoplasia similar to human subtype 2A in a dog: Medullary thyroid carcinoma, bilateral pheochromocytoma and parathyroid adenoma. Open Veterinary Journal. 2016;**6**(3):165-171

[29] Piñeyro P, Vieson MD, Ramos-Vara JA, Moon-Larson M, Saunders G. Histopathological and immunohistochemical findings of primary and metastatic medullary thyroid carcinoma in a young dog. JVS. 2014;**15**(3):449-453

[30] Schmid KW. Histopathology of C cells and medullary thyroid carcinoma. In: Raue F, editor. Medullary Thyroid Carcinoma: Biology–Management–Treatment. Cham: Springer International Publishing; 2015. pp. 41-60

[31] Gibbons PM, Garner MM, Kiupel M. Morphological and immunohistochemical characterization of spontaneous thyroid gland neoplasms in guinea pigs (*Cavia porcellus*). Veterinary Pathology. 2012;**50**(2):334-342

[32] Iwamoto Y, Kassai T. Two cases of feline thyroid carcinoma. Journal of Animal Clinical Medicine. 2017;**26**(2):76-80

[33] Saulez MN, Viljoen A, Kafka U, Rubio-Martinez L, van Wilpe E, Steyl J. The use of nuclear imaging for a mixed C cell microfollicular carcinoma of the thyroid gland in a mature horse. Equine Veterinary Education. 2013;**25**(3):118-125

[34] Vítovec J. Epithelial thyroid tumors in cows. Veterinary Pathology. 1976;**13**(6):401-408

[35] Harmon BG, Kelley LC. Immunohistochemistry of ultimobranchial thyroid carcinomas in seven slaughtered cows and one bull. Journal of Veterinary Diagnostic Investigation. 2001;**13**(2):101-105

[36] Brandão J, Manickam B, Blas-Machado U, Cohen E, Mejia-Fava J, Divers S, et al. Productive thyroid follicular carcinoma in a wild barred owl (Strix varia). Journal of Veterinary Diagnostic Investigation. 2012;**24**(6):1145-1150

[37] Bartsch R, Brinkmann B, Jahnke G, Laube B, Lohmann R, Michaelsen S, et al. Human relevance of follicular thyroid tumors in rodents caused by non-genotoxic substances. Regulatory Toxicology and Pharmacology. 2018;**98**:199-208

[38] Wills TB, Bohn AA, Finch NP, Harris SP, Caplazi P. Thyroid follicular adenocarcinoma in a ferret. Veterinary Clinical Pathology. 2005;**34**(4):405-408

[39] Fox JG, Dangler CA, Snyder SB, Richard MJ, Thilsted JP. C-cell carcinoma (medullary thyroid carcinoma) associated with multiple endocrine neoplasms in a ferret (*Mustela putorius*). Veterinary Pathology. 2000;**37**(3):278-282

[40] Fournie JW, Wolfe MJ, Wolf JC, Courtney LA, Johnson RD, Hawkins WE. Diagnostic criteria for proliferative thyroid lesions in bony fishes. Toxicologic Pathology. 2005;**33**(5):540-551

[41] Shimamura M, Shibusawa N, KurashigeT,MussazhanovaZ,MatsuzakiH, Nakashima M, et al. Mouse models of sporadic thyroid cancer derived from BRAFV600E alone or in combination with PTEN haploinsufficiency under physiologic TSH levels. PLoS One. 2018;**13**(8):e0201365

[42] Davis BW, Ostrander EA. Domestic dogs and cancer research: A breed-based genomics approach. ILAR Journal. 2014;**55**(1):59-68

[43] Frantz LAF, Bradley DG, Larson G, Orlando L. Animal domestication in the era of ancient genomics. Nature Reviews. Genetics. 2020;**21**(8):449-460

[44] Boge GS, Moldal ER, Dimopoulou M, Skjerve E, Bergström A. Breed susceptibility for common surgically treated orthopaedic diseases in 12 dog breeds. Acta Veterinaria Scandinavica. 2019;**61**(1):19

[45] Edmunds GL, Smalley MJ, Beck S, Errington RJ, Gould S, Winter H, et al. Dog breeds and body conformations with predisposition to osteosarcoma in the UK: A case-control study. Canine Medicine and Genetics. 2021;**8**(1):2

[46] Farrell LL, Schoenebeck JJ, Wiener P, Clements DN, Summers KM. The challenges of pedigree dog health: Approaches to combating inherited disease. Canine Genetics and Epidemiology. 2015;**2**(1):3

Chapter 4

The Molecular Basis for Radioiodine Therapy

Gerardo Hernán Carro and Juan Pablo Nicola

Abstract

Radioactive iodine (radioiodine) therapy is a standard and effective therapeutic approach for high-risk differentiated thyroid carcinomas, based on the unique ability of the thyroid follicular cell to accumulate iodide through the sodium/iodide symporter (NIS). However, a recurrent limitation of radioiodine therapy is the development of radioiodine-refractory differentiated thyroid carcinomas, which are associated with a worse prognosis. Loss of radioiodine accumulation in thyroid carcinomas has been attributed to cell dedifferentiation, resulting in reduced NIS expression and NIS intracellular retention involving transcriptional and posttranscriptional or posttranslational mechanisms, respectively. Emerging therapies targeting the oncogene-activated signal pathways potentially involved in thyroid carcinogenesis have been able to recover radioiodine accumulation in radioiodine-refractory tumors, which constitutes the rationale of redifferentiation therapies. Here, we will comprehensively discuss the molecular mechanisms underlying radioiodine therapy, refractoriness to radioiodine therapy in differentiated thyroid carcinomas, and novel strategies for restoring radioiodine accumulation in radioiodine-refractory thyroid carcinomas.

Keywords: differentiated thyroid cancer, sodium/iodide symporter, radioiodine therapy, radioiodine-refractory thyroid cancer, redifferentiation therapy

1. Introduction

The ability of the thyroid follicular cell to accumulate iodide constitutes the cornerstone for diagnostic scintigraphy and therapy for hyperfunctioning thyroid tissue, as well as for differentiated thyroid carcinoma and their metastases after thyroidectomy [1]. Radioactive iodine (radioiodine) administration used in thyroid tissue remnant ablation after thyroidectomy and adjuvant therapy in metastatic differentiated thyroid carcinomas has been possibly the most successful internal radiation therapy ever designed. In patients with high-risk differentiated thyroid carcinomas, retrospective studies have demonstrated that the ability of tumor cells to accumulate radioiodine is the best indicator of disease-free and of overall survival [2].

Currently, thyroid hormone withdrawal and recombinant thyrotropin-stimulated radioiodine adjuvant therapy are considered in intermediate-risk carcinomas and are routinely recommended for high-risk differentiated thyroid carcinomas after total thyroidectomy [3]. However, differentiated thyroid tumors often exhibit reduced (or even undetectable) radioiodine accumulation, compared with normal thyroid tissue, and are diagnosed as cold nodules using thyroid scintigraphy. Despite this reduction, over 70% of differentiated thyroid carcinomas accumulate radioiodine to some extent, which is still sufficient to achieve adequate radioiodine accumulation for treatment. Unfortunately, 30% of metastatic differentiated thyroid tumors completely lose their ability to accumulate iodide, with this percentage increasing up to 70% when the oncogene BRAFV600E is present. This causes thyroid tumors to become refractory to radioiodine therapy and is associated with a poor outcome. Patients with thyroid cancer metastases that accumulate iodide show a survival rate at 10 years of ~60%, while survival is drastically reduced to ~10% in patients with radioiodine refractory metastases [4]. Therefore, a better understanding of the biological mechanisms leading to differentiated thyroid carcinoma resistance to radioiodine therapy will certainly have major implications for its treatment [5].

The clinical experience of radioiodine theranostic in the management of differentiated thyroid cancer has opened up a complete new field related to developing strategies to extend this promising approach to non-thyroidal cancers. Although, in addition to thyroid cancer, functional endogenous radioiodine accumulation has only been observed in breast and ovarian cancer [6, 7], this could be key for radioiodine being used as an effective therapeutic tool. The ectopic induction of radioiodine accumulation using gene transfer has paved the way for the development of new therapeutic strategies to treat tumors with radioiodine, as in differentiated thyroid cancer. Since a pioneering study successfully induced iodide accumulation in malignant transformed thyroid cells that did not accumulate iodide, thereby rendering them sensitive to radioiodine treatment [8], a large body of evidence has shown the feasibility of inducing radioiodine accumulation in several cancer cell lines [9, 10].

2. Iodide metabolism in the thyroid follicular cell

Iodine is an essential constituent of thyroid hormones. Therefore, a fundamental condition for normal thyroid hormonogenesis is that iodide—an extremely scarce environmental micronutrient—should be made available in sufficient amounts to the thyroid follicular cells (also known as thyrocytes), which have developed a remarkably efficient and specialized iodide-handling system. Under physiological conditions, the thyroid gland accumulates iodide al concentrations up to 40 times those in the plasma. The sodium/iodide symporter (NIS) is the key plasma membrane glycoprotein, which is located at the basolateral surface of the thyroid follicular cell that mediates active iodide transport from the bloodstream to the thyroid follicular cells in the first step and the rate-limiting step of thyroid hormonogenesis [11]. The carboxy-terminus of the protein, which is oriented toward the cytoplasm, contains specific sorting and retention signals required for NIS expression at the basolateral plasma membrane [12–15]. NIS-mediated active iodide transport is electrogenic and couples the inward translocation of one iodide ion against its electrochemical gradient to the inward transport of two sodium ions down its electrochemical gradient, generated by the sodium/potassium ATPase [16]. Remarkably, NIS transports iodide efficiently at the submicromolar concentrations found in the bloodstream, by taking advantage of the physiological sodium concentration [17]. Therefore, the mechanism of NIS-mediated iodide transport seems to be an evolutionary adaptation to the scant amount of iodide in the environment.

In addition to the different radioiodide isotopes, NIS can translocate a variety of clinically relevant radionuclide substrates. These include ^{99m}Tc-pertechnectate or ^{18}F-tetrafluoroborate, which facilitates noninvasive diagnostic imaging, and also ^{188}Re-perrhenate, which allows therapeutic destruction of tumor tissue through the radionuclide accumulation of NIS-expressing cells and the bystander effect induced by the crossfire effect of beta emission [10].

Underscoring the significance of NIS for thyroid physiology, several naturally occurring loss-of-function NIS variants have been identified as causes of the uncommon autosomal recessive disorder iodide transport defect, which results in dyshormonogenic congenital hypothyroidism due to insufficient iodide availability for thyroid hormonogenesis [9]. Moreover, a recent study speculated that pathogenic variants may exist in yet to be discovered thyroid-specific genes and are likely to be required for NIS-mediated iodide transport in the thyroid follicular cell [18]. In line with this hypothesis, the KCNQ1/KCNE2 potassium channel has been shown to be required for adequate NIS-mediated iodide accumulation in the thyroid tissue [19, 20]. The detailed functional characterization of loss-of-function NIS variants identified in patients has provided mechanistic information about the transporter. Remarkably, several amino acid residues have been identified as being critical for substrate binding, specificity, and stoichiometry, as well as for folding and plasma membrane targeting [21–28].

Once iodide has reached the cytosol of the thyroid follicular cells, the iodide is then handled by a sophisticated thyroid-specific iodine-metabolizing machinery that covalently incorporates (also named organification) iodine into tyrosine residues of thyroglobulin, which permits further thyroid hormone synthesis [29]. Significantly, the normal function of this iodide-metabolizing machinery is not only critical for thyroid hormonogenesis, but also for successful radioiodine ablation of cancer cells, as the covalent incorporation of radioiodine into thyroglobulin increases the residence time of the radioisotope.

3. Radioiodine therapy

Radioiodine therapy relies on the unique property of the thyroid follicular cell to transport and incorporate iodide into thyroglobulin, a feature that is maintained in a subgroup of differentiated thyroid carcinomas. Postoperative radioiodine administration can be used to destroy presumably benign residual thyroid tissue (remnant ablation), to destroy suspected but not identified remaining disease (adjuvant treatment), and to destroy known residual or recurrent disease (treatment) [30]. Until recently, most patients with differentiated thyroid carcinoma received postoperative radioiodine therapy, constituting a standard of care. Nowadays, radioiodine therapy has been personalized based on the risk of recurrence stratification and the prognostic indicators obtained during thyroidectomy and also on the findings of postoperative neck ultrasound and serum thyroglobulin levels. Radioiodine therapy is currently exceptionally recommended in patients with low-risk thyroid cancers, which represents the majority of patients with thyroid cancer.

Radioiodine is administered following thyrotropin (TSH) stimulation, the primary regulator of NIS expression in the thyroid follicular cell at both the transcriptional and posttranscriptional levels. TSH stimulation is achieved either by long-term withdrawal of thyroid hormone replacement treatment or after recombinant human TSH treatment. The use of recombinant human TSH avoids symptoms of hypothyroidism, thereby improving the quality of life of the patients [31]. Restriction of dietary iodine is often recommended, and iodinated radiocontrast agents should be excluded before radioiodine scanning or treatment of differentiated thyroid carcinomas to avoid isotopic dilution, thus possibly improving radioiodine therapy efficacy [32].

Papillary thyroid carcinoma, the most prevalent form of the disease and accounting for approximately 85% of differentiated thyroid carcinomas, includes several tumor subtypes of which ~70% have mutually exclusive mutations of gene-encoding effectors of the mitogen-activated protein kinase (MAPK) signal pathway [33]. The papillary thyroid cancer genome atlas has revealed that the main genomic alterations include point mutations in the proto-oncogenes BRAF and (N, H, or K) RAS and also chromosomal rearrangements involving the proto-oncogenes RET and NTRK [34]. Significantly, BRAFV600E-harboring papillary thyroid carcinomas frequently have a poor response to radioiodine therapy [35]. Related to this, their refractoriness to radioiodine appears to be due to the strong BRAFV600E-triggered MAPK-dependent transcriptional program suppressing (or even abolishing) the expression of genes involved in iodide uptake and metabolism, which are hallmarks of the differentiated state of thyroid follicular cells. In contrast, RAS-mutated papillary thyroid carcinomas show a low MAPK-dependent transcriptional program (due to negative feedback regulation), retaining the expression of iodine-metabolism genes, and are usually radioiodine-avid [36]. Low frequency types of differentiated thyroid carcinomas, such as Hürthle-cell carcinomas and poorly differentiated thyroid carcinomas, are particularly refractory to radioiodine therapy.

Since, as mentioned above, BRAFV600E is frequently associated with decreased responsiveness to radioiodine, an emerging clinically relevant question is whether genetic markers can reliably predict the radioiodine refractoriness of thyroid carcinomas [37]. Indeed, recent studies have demonstrated that ~70% of patients with metastatic papillary thyroid cancer carrying the oncogene BRAFV600E do not demonstrate any radioiodine uptake, with this percentage increasing up to 97% when BRAFV600E is associated with mutations in the promoter of the Telomerase Reverse Transcriptase (TERT) [38, 39]. However, a subset of BRAFV600E-carrying papillary thyroid carcinomas does respond to radioiodide therapy [36]. Significantly, the BRAFV600E-containing papillary thyroid tumors that showed better responses to radioiodine therapy also revealed a relatively preserved expression of thyroid differentiation genes, and a higher expression of microRNAs targeting the transforming growth factor β (TGFβ) signaling pathway, which when activated repressed thyroid-specific gene expression [40].

4. Radioiodine-refractory thyroid cancer

Approximately 80 years after the first clinical use of radioiodine therapy for the diagnosis and treatment of differentiated thyroid cancer [41], radioiodine therapy is still the first choice of treatment after thyroidectomy for primary and metastatic differentiated thyroid carcinomas. However, 30% of metastatic differentiated thyroid tumors show dedifferentiation and lose their ability to accumulate radioiodine, thus making adjuvant treatment with radioiodine ineffective (radioiodine-refractory) [42]. Current therapeutic strategies for symptomatic radioiodine-refractory thyroid cancers include the implementation of local therapy whenever possible. However, in the case of diffuse significant progression of distant metastatic disease, systemic therapy is currently based on anti-angiogenic multi-targeted tyrosine kinase inhibitors [43]. The two multi-targeted tyrosine kinase inhibitors sorafenib and lenvatinib have been approved by regulatory authorities for use in radioiodine-refractory differentiated thyroid carcinomas [44, 45]. These agents have shown promising results with a significant improvement of median progression-free survival over placebo, but generally with similar overall survival. More recently, novel highly selective inhibitors targeting oncogenic chromosomal rearrangements involving the proto-oncogenes RET and NTRK have been approved for clinical use in radioiodine-refractory differentiated thyroid carcinomas [46, 47]. Therefore, the presence of druggable oncogenes should be screened in patients with metastatic disease, and whenever present, a selective inhibitor might be considered.

The underlying molecular basis for the loss of radioiodine accumulation in radioiodine-refractory metastatic thyroid carcinomas is thyroid dedifferentiation, which results in a decreased expression of the genes involved in the iodide metabolism. Radioiodine therapy effectivity is ultimately dependent on functional NIS expression at the plasma membrane of the thyroid tumor cells, as deficient radioiodide accumulation is the major cause of treatment failure [5]. However, NIS gene expression is frequently downregulated in differentiated thyroid cancer compared with normal thyroid tissue or even totally silenced as evidenced in poorly differentiated carcinomas. Multiple transcriptional and posttranscriptional mechanisms have been postulated to explain NIS gene repression in thyroid tumors, including transcriptional repression of the transcription factor Pax8 that regulates NIS gene transcriptional expression, and by TGFB1-induced activation of SMAD signaling leading to NOX4-dependent ROS production, which in turn impairs Pax8-dependent NIS gene expression [48, 49]. Immunohistochemical studies have revealed that NIS is frequently expressed (or even overexpressed) at different levels in differentiated thyroid carcinomas compared with adjacent normal tissue [50]. However, NIS expression is mainly located in intracellular compartments, indicating that a posttranslational mechanism is involved in radioiodide resistance due to defective NIS expression at the plasma membrane [51, 52]. Significantly, loss-of-function NIS variants have not been identified in either benign cold thyroid nodules or thyroid tumors [53, 54], demonstrating that the intracellular retention of NIS is not caused by structural defects, as reported in patients with dyshormonogenic congenital hypothyroidism. Therefore, the paradoxical observation of reduced radioiodine uptake and intracellularly retained NIS protein expression highlights the importance of elucidating the posttranslational mechanisms regulating NIS plasma membrane expression.

The pituitary tumor-transforming gene (PTTG) binding factor (PBF) has been reported as being an NIS-interacting protein involved in NIS intracellular retention in thyroid cancer, as ectopic PBF overexpression results in reduced iodide accumulation caused by NIS endocytosis from the plasma membrane [55]. The phosphorylation of the PBF residue Tyr-174 is required for PBF-mediated NIS endocytosis, as PP1-inhibited Src kinase activity restores iodide accumulation in thyroid cancer cell lines [56]. Moreover, chemical inhibition of the NIS-interacting protein valosin-containing protein (VCP), a principal component of the endoplasmic reticulum-associated degradation protein quality control process involved in NIS proteolysis, increases NIS expression at the plasma membrane and radioiodide accumulation in thyroid cancer models [57]. Recently, high-throughput drug screening has revealed multiple cellular processes that are central to NIS regulation, including proteasomal degradation and autophagy, which can be drugged to enhance radioiodide uptake [58]. Moreover, functional defects in the glycosylphosphatidylinositol (GPI) transamidase complex due to $BRAF^{V600E}$-triggered PIGU repression cause partially glycosylated NIS molecules to be retained in the endoplasmic reticulum, probably due to a deficiency in an unidentified GPI-anchored protein that is necessary for proper NIS anterograde plasma membrane transport [59].

Constitutive activation of mitogen-activated protein kinase (MAPK) signaling induces a partial to complete loss of differentiation in thyroid cancers. In agreement, *in vitro* studies have revealed that BRAFV600E impairs NIS expression, thereby reducing iodide uptake [60]. In patients, BRAFV600E expression in papillary thyroid carcinoma was correlated with radioiodine-refractory recurrences and defective NIS expression or intracellular retention [61]. In line with this, transgenic mice expressing the oncogene BRAFV600E in thyroid follicular cells developed papillary thyroid tumors, with these tumors neither concentrating radioiodine nor responding to radioiodine therapy [62]. Interestingly, the blockage of BRAFV600E kinase activity with either the BRAFV600E-selective ATP competitive inhibitor PLX4720, a vemurafenib progenitor, or further downstream with the allosteric MEK 1/2 kinase inhibitor selumetinib, restored thyroid-specific gene expression (including NIS) and radioiodine incorporation into these tumors, which rendered them susceptible to therapeutic doses of radioiodine [62].

When used as single agents, vemurafenib and selumetinib are comparatively ineffective inhibitors of BRAFV600E-driven thyroid cancer. Although they are potent inhibitors of MAPK-ERK signaling in thyroid cancer, this inhibition is followed by a strong rebound effect that reactivates ERK signaling. Blockage of ERK-dependent negative feedback mechanisms increases the expression of the tyrosine kinase HER3, with its activation after dimerization with HER2 by the autocrine-secreted ligand neuregulin leading to ERK activation involving CRAF signaling [63]. Significantly, the allosteric MEK 1/2 inhibitor CH5126766, when bound to the protein, impairs its phosphorylation by upstream (A, B, or C) RAF kinases and reduces reactivation of ERK signaling, which overcomes the adaptive resistance of BRAFV600E-promoted thyroid cancer to MAPK inhibitors and markedly enhances the effectiveness of radioiodine therapy [64].

5. Redifferentiation therapy

Recent progress in understanding the molecular mechanisms that repress functional NIS expression has identified possibilities of new therapeutic approaches, which may expand the application of radioiodine therapy to radioiodine-refractory thyroid cancers. Indeed, some emerging therapies using MAPK signal small-molecule inhibitors, which are still in the clinical phase of study, have shown promising effects by restoring radioiodine accumulation in radioiodine-refractory differentiated thyroid cancer metastasis (redifferentiation therapy) [65].

Encouraging preclinical data, suggesting that MAPK signaling inhibition in BRAFV600E-induced thyroid cancer mouse models partially restores radioiodine accumulation [62, 64], has prompted pilot clinical studies in patients with thyroid cancer metastases resistant to radioiodide. In the first pilot clinical trial, selumetinib treatment restored iodide uptake at metastatic sites in 12 out of 20 patients with advanced radioiodine-refractory papillary thyroid cancer, and with eight of these attaining the predefined dosimetry threshold to enable radioiodine therapy with remarkable clinical responses: five of which had partial responses and with the other three having stable disease at 6 months after therapy [66]. Significantly, the therapeutic benefit of selumetinib was dependent on the mutation landscape, as all five patients carrying NRASQ61R/K, but only one of nine patients carrying BRAFV600E, redifferentiated sufficiently to be able to receive radioiodine therapy [66].

The BRAFV600E inhibitor dabrafenib was evaluated in patients with BRAFV600E-containing advanced radioiodine-refractory metastatic papillary thyroid cancer [67]. Dabrafenib treatment restored iodide uptake at metastatic sites in six out of 10 patients, and all these six patients were then treated with radioiodine, leading to a partial response and stable disease in two and four patients, respectively, at 3 months after therapy [67]. In a more recent pilot clinical trial, another BRAF inhibitor, vemurafenib, was evaluated in patients with BRAFV600E-containing advanced radioiodine-refractory metastatic papillary thyroid cancer [68]. Vemurafenib treatment restored or increased radioiodine accumulation in at least one metastatic lesion in six out of 10 patients. Of these, four patients attained the predefined dosimetry threshold and received radioiodide therapy, resulting in disease-free progression, with two confirmed partial responses and two with stable disease at 6 months after therapy [68]. Significantly, a transcriptomic analysis of tumor biopsy revealed that vemurafenib treatment reduced the MAPK pathway transcriptional output and induced thyroid differentiation markers [68].

In an interesting retrospective review of clinical data, six patients with radioiodine-refractory thyroid carcinomas received mutation-guided redifferentiation therapy [69]. Patients with NRASQ61K/R-harboring tumors were treated with the MEK inhibitor trametinib, and those with BRAFV600E received a combination of BRAF and MAPK inhibitors (dabrafenib and trametinib, or vemurafenib and cobimetinib). Redifferentiation therapy restored radioiodine accumulation in one of the three patients with NRASQ61K, and in all three patients with BRAFV600E. Radioiodine therapy was applied to these four patients, with three achieving a partial response and one having a stable disease under a median follow-up of 16.6 months [69]. Significantly, this study suggests that the mutation-guided MAPK pathway combined inhibition is a promising strategy to redifferentiate BRAFV600E radioiodine-refractory thyroid carcinomas, thereby rendering them suitable for radioiodine therapy.

Very recently, the results were published of the first large-scale phase 3 clinical trial conducted to evaluate the clinical benefit of adding selumetinib to adjuvant radioiodine therapy in patients with a high-risk of persistent disease or disease recurrence following initial total thyroidectomy [70]. Of the 233 patients enrolled, 97% of the placebo group and 83% of the selumetinib group completed the treatment. The complete response rate analysis at 18 months revealed no statistically significant improvement in response to selumetinib therapy compared with placebo.

The adaptive resistance to MAPK inhibitors driven by neuregulin-dependent HER3/HER2 activation observed in BRAF-mutated thyroid cancers led to testing the strategy of combining MAPK inhibitors with EGF receptor (HER) inhibitors. Significantly, the HER kinase inhibitor lapatinib prevented MAPK rebound and overcame BRAFV600E thyroid cancer cell resistance to MAPK inhibitors [63]. Similarly, in BRAFV600E expressing human thyroid cancer cell lines, the combination of lapatinib with dabrafenib or selumetinib increased radioiodine accumulation [71]. Based on the abovementioned preclinical data, a recent small pilot clinical trial assessed vemurafenib in combination with ErbB3 targeting of monoclonal antibody CDX-3379 in radioiodine-refractory metastatic thyroid cancer carrying BRAFV600E [72]. This combined therapy increased radioiodine accumulation in five out of six patients, of which four patients had a sufficient reaction to warrant radioiodine therapy. At 6 months post-therapy, two of these patients achieved a confirmed partial response [72].

Recently, Saqsena et al. [73] investigated the impact of the SWItch/Sucrose Non-Fermentable (SWI/SNF) chromatin remodeling complex on BRAFV600E-driven thyroid cancer differentiation. Mechanistically, the functional loss of different

SWI/SNF subunits reduced the expression of thyroid differentiation markers by repressing chromatin accessibility to the gene encoding different transcription factors required for expression of genes regulating iodide transport and metabolism. Importantly, SWI/SNF loss promoted resistance to MAPK inhibitor–based redifferentiation therapies, reducing the effectiveness of radioiodine treatment [73]. Moreover, the preclinical data suggest that mutations affecting individual SWI/SNF complex subunits should be investigated as potential markers of resistance to redifferentiation strategies, as patients with radioiodine-refractory tumors carrying biallelic mutations in the SWI/SNF complex genes ARID1A, ARID2, or SMARCB1 failed to show a clinically significant restoration of radioiodine incorporation in response to MAPK pathway inhibition [72, 73].

The development of well-tolerated systemic therapies that selectively target oncogenic chromosomal rearrangements involved in thyroid carcinogenesis has extended the landscape of therapeutic opportunities in radioiodine-refractory thyroid carcinomas [46, 47]. Recently, different clinical case reports have revealed that the selective NTRK inhibitor larotrectinib restored radioiodine accumulation in radioiodine-refractory lung metastases harboring the NTRK fusions EML4-NTRK3, TPR-NTRK1, ETV6-NTRK3, and TPM3-NTRK1 [74–76]. Likewise, the selective RET inhibitor selpercantinib restored radioiodine accumulation in radioiodine-refractory lung metastases harboring RET fusions CCDC6-RET and NCOA4-RET [75, 77]. Moreover, a recent report presented the case of a pediatric patient with a TPM3-NTRK1 fusion-positive lung metastatic papillary thyroid carcinoma, who received redifferentiation therapy with larotrectinib as a neoadjuvant systemic approach, before the initial dose of radioiodine [78].

6. Conclusions

Radioiodine accumulation in the thyroid tissue has been exploited in clinical medicine in the diagnosis and treatment of thyroid pathologies for several decades, even before the molecular characterization of the mechanism mediating iodide accumulation. Since the cloning of NIS, significant progress has been made in understanding the mechanisms mediating the resistance to radioiodine therapy, with the efficacy of the therapy having been shown to be directly related to the therapeutic dose of radiation delivered to tumor cells [79]. From a therapeutic perspective, improving radioiodine therapy for thyroid cancer is a priority for developing strategies aimed not only at enhancing radioiodine accumulation but also for promoting efficient radioiodine organification for its retention inside thyroid tumor cells, in order to improve radiation dose delivery to provide better treatment efficacy. Significantly, experimental models have revealed that phosphoinositide 3-kinase (PI3K) inhibitors seem to prolong radioiodine retention in thyroid cells [80].

The understanding of the molecular events involved in the biology of thyroid cancer has rapidly expanded the therapeutic landscape for the treatment of iodine-refractory thyroid cancer. Redifferentiation therapy has emerged as an attractive alternative in the clinical management of radioiodine-refractory thyroid carcinomas, but the promising clinical data are still preliminary. However, monotherapy with MAPK inhibitors only increases iodide accumulation in a marginal fraction of patients with metastatic thyroid cancers expressing BRAFV600E, probably due to incomplete MAPK signaling inhibition, thus suggesting that profound inhibition of MAPK signaling is required for treating these tumors effectively. The identification of novel small-molecule inhibitors exhibiting a stronger and sustained inhibition of MAPK signaling may provide novel alternatives for maximizing the response to radioiodine therapy.

An emerging topic is the value of genetic marker-based precision management of radioiodine therapy in thyroid cancer. The co-occurrence of TERT promoter mutations in BRAFV600E-carrying recurrent papillary thyroid carcinomas is associated with loss of radioiodine accumulation. Moreover, the functional loss of SWI/SNF subunits may mediate resistance to redifferentiation therapies and might serve as biomarkers for identifying patients who will not benefit from this therapy. Although large clinical trials are necessary to validate this hypothesis, the presence of deleterious SWI/SNF subunit lesions may prompt physicians to consider treatments other than radioiodide.

Acknowledgements

We are grateful to Dr. Ana María Masini-Repiso (National University of Córdoba, Argentina) for critical reading of the manuscript. This work was supported by Fondo para la Investigación Científica y Tecnológica - Agencia Nacional de Promoción Científica y Tecnológica (grants number PICT-2018-1596, PICT-2019-1772, PIDC-2019-0007, and PICT-2021-0005).

Conflict of interest

The authors declare no conflict of interest.

Author details

Gerardo Hernán Carro[1,2] and Juan Pablo Nicola[1,2]*

1 Faculty of Chemical Sciences, Department of Clinical Biochemistry, National University of Córdoba, Córdoba, Argentina

2 Clinical Biochemistry and Immunology Research Center, National Scientific and Technical Research Council (CIBICI-CONICET), Córdoba, Argentina

*Address all correspondence to: juan.nicola@unc.edu.ar

References

[1] Schlumberger M, Leboulleux S. Current practice in patients with differentiated thyroid cancer. Nature Reviews. Endocrinology. 2021;**17**:176-188

[2] Tuttle RM, Ahuja S, Avram AM, Bernet VJ, Bourguet P, Daniels GH, et al. Controversies, Consensus, and Collaboration in the Use of (131) I Therapy in Differentiated Thyroid Cancer: A Joint Statement from the American Thyroid Association, the European Association of Nuclear Medicine, the Society of Nuclear Medicine and Molecular Imaging, and the European Thyroid Association. Thyroid. 2019;**29**:461-470

[3] Haugen BR, Alexander EK, Bible KC, Doherty GM, Mandel SJ, Nikiforov YE, et al. 2015 American Thyroid Association Management Guidelines for Adult Patients with Thyroid Nodules and Differentiated Thyroid Cancer. Thyroid. 2016;**26**:1-133

[4] Durante C, Haddy N, Baudin E, Leboulleux S, Hartl D, Travagli JP, et al. Long-term outcome of 444 patients with distant metastases from papillary and follicular thyroid carcinoma: Benefits and limits of radioiodine therapy. The Journal of Clinical Endocrinology and Metabolism. 2006;**91**:2892-2899

[5] Schlumberger M, Lacroix L, Russo D, Filetti S, Bidart JM. Defects in iodide metabolism in thyroid cancer and implications for the follow-up and treatment of patients. Nature Clinical Practice. Endocrinology & Metabolism. 2007;**3**:260-269

[6] Tazebay UH, Wapnir IL, Levy O, Dohan O, Zuckier LS, Zhao QH, et al. The mammary gland iodide transporter is expressed during lactation and in breast cancer. Nature Medicine. 2000;**6**:871-878

[7] Riesco-Eizaguirre G, Leoni SG, Mendiola M, Estevez-Cebrero MA, Gallego MI, Redondo A, et al. NIS mediates iodide uptake in the female reproductive tract and is a poor prognostic factor in ovarian cancer. The Journal of Clinical Endocrinology and Metabolism. 2014;**99**:E1199-E1208

[8] Shimura H, Haraguchi K, Miyazaki A, Endo T, Onaya T. Iodide uptake and experimental 131I therapy in transplanted undifferentiated thyroid cancer cells expressing the Na+/I- symporter gene. Endocrinology. 1997;**138**:4493-4496

[9] Ravera S, Reyna-Neyra A, Ferrandino G, Amzel LM, Carrasco N. The sodium/iodide symporter (NIS): Molecular physiology and preclinical and clinical applications. Annual Review of Physiology. 2017;**79**:261-289

[10] Kitzberger C, Spellerberg R, Morath V, Schwenk N, Schmohl KA, Schug C, et al. The sodium iodide symporter (NIS) as theranostic gene: Its emerging role in new imaging modalities and non-viral gene therapy. EJNMMI Research. 2022;**12**:25

[11] Martín M, Geysels RC, Peyret V, Bernal Barquero CE, Masini-Repiso AM, Nicola JP. Implications of Na+/I- symporter transport to the plasma membrane for thyroid hormonogenesis and radioiodide therapy. Journal of Endocrinology Society. 2019;**3**:222-234

[12] Martin M, Modenutti CP, Peyret V, Geysels RC, Darrouzet E, Pourcher T, et al. A carboxy-terminal monoleucine-based motif participates

in the basolateral targeting of the Na+/I- symporter. Endocrinology. 2019;**160**:156-168

[13] Martín M, Salleron L, Peyret V, Geysels RC, Darrouzet E, Lindenthal S, et al. The PDZ protein SCRIB regulates sodium/iodide symporter (NIS) expression at the basolateral plasma membrane. The FASEB Journal. 2021;**35**:e21681

[14] Martín M, Modenutti CP, Gil Rosas ML, Peyret V, Geysels RC, Bernal Barquero CE, et al. A Novel SLC5A5 variant reveals the crucial role of kinesin light chain 2 in thyroid hormonogenesis. The Journal of Clinical Endocrinology and Metabolism. 2021;**106**:1867-1881

[15] Koumarianou P, Fernandez-Mendez C, Fajardo-Delgado D, Mielu LM, Santisteban P, de la Vieja A. Basolateral sorting of the sodium iodide symporter NIS is mediated by AP-1 clathrin adaptor complexes. Thyroid. 2022. DOI: 10.1089/thy.2022.0163 [In press]

[16] Ravera S, Quick M, Nicola JP, Carrasco N, Amzel LM. Beyond non-integer Hill coefficients: A novel approach to analyzing binding data, applied to Na+-driven transporters. The Journal of General Physiology. 2015;**145**:555-563

[17] Nicola JP, Carrasco N, Amzel LM. Physiological sodium concentrations enhance the iodide affinity of the Na+/I- symporter. Nature Communications. 2014;**5**:3948

[18] Bernal Barquero CE, Geysels RC, Jacques V, Carro GH, Martín M, Peyret V, et al. Targeted next-generation sequencing of congenital hypothyroidism-causative genes reveals unexpected thyroglobulin gene variants in patients with iodide transport defect. International Journal of Molecular Sciences. 2022;**23**:1825955

[19] Purtell K, Paroder-Belenitsky M, Reyna-Neyra A, Nicola JP, Koba W, Fine E, et al. The KCNQ1-KCNE2 K+ channel is required for adequate thyroid I- uptake. The FASEB Journal. 2012;**26**:3252-3259

[20] Frohlich H, Boini KM, Seebohm G, Strutz-Seebohm N, Ureche ON, Foller M, et al. Hypothyroidism of gene-targeted mice lacking Kcnq1. Pflügers Archiv. 2011;**461**:45-52

[21] Nicola JP, Reyna-Neyra A, Saenger P, Rodriguez-Buritica DF, Gamez Godoy JD, Muzumdar R, et al. Sodium/Iodide symporter mutant V270E causes stunted growth but no cognitive deficiency. The Journal of Clinical Endocrinology and Metabolism. 2015;**100**:E1353-E1361

[22] Paroder V, Nicola JP, Ginter CS, Carrasco N. The iodide-transport-defect-causing mutation R124H: A delta-amino group at position 124 is critical for maturation and trafficking of the Na+/I- symporter. Journal of Cell Science. 2013;**126**:3305-3313

[23] Li W, Nicola JP, Amzel LM, Carrasco N. Asn441 plays a key role in folding and function of the Na+/I- symporter (NIS). The FASEB Journal. 2013;**27**:3229-3238

[24] Paroder-Belenitsky M, Maestas MJ, Dohan O, Nicola JP, Reyna-Neyra A, Follenzi A, et al. Mechanism of anion selectivity and stoichiometry of the Na+/I- symporter (NIS). Proceedings of the National Academy of Sciences of the United States of America. 2011;**108**:17933-17938

[25] De la Vieja A, Reed MD, Ginter CS, Carrasco N. Amino acid residues in transmembrane segment IX of the Na+/I- symporter play a role in its Na+ dependence and are critical for transport activity. The Journal of Biological Chemistry. 2007;**282**:25290-25298

[26] Geysels RC, Bernal Barquero CE, Martin M, Peyret V, Nocent M, Sobrero G, et al. Silent but not harmless: A synonymous SLC5A5 gene variant leading to dyshormonogenic congenital hypothyroidism. Front Endocrinol (Lausanne). 2022;**13**:868891

[27] Bernal Barquero CE, Martín M, Geysels RC, Peyret V, Papendieck P, Masini-Repiso AM, et al. An intramolecular ionic interaction linking defective sodium/iodide symporter transport to the plasma membrane and dyshormonogenic congenital hypothyroidism. Thyroid. 2022;**32**:19-27

[28] Martin M, Bernal Barquero CE, Geysels RC, Papendieck P, Peyret V, Masini-Repiso AM, et al. Novel sodium/iodide symporter compound heterozygous pathogenic variants causing dyshormonogenic congenital hypothyroidism. Thyroid. 2019;**29**:1023-1026

[29] Tosatto L, Coscia F. A glance at post-translational modifications of human thyroglobulin: Potential impact on function and pathogenesis. European Thyroid Journal. 2022;**11**:e220046

[30] Tuttle RM. Distinguishing remnant ablation from adjuvant treatment in differentiated thyroid cancer. The Lancet Diabetes and Endocrinology. 2019;**7**:7-8

[31] Schlumberger M, Ricard M, De Pouvourville G, Pacini F. How the availability of recombinant human TSH has changed the management of patients who have thyroid cancer. Nature Clinical Practice. Endocrinology & Metabolism. 2007;**3**:641-650

[32] Sawka AM, Ibrahim-Zada I, Galacgac P, Tsang RW, Brierley JD, Ezzat S, et al. Dietary iodine restriction in preparation for radioactive iodine treatment or scanning in well-differentiated thyroid cancer: A systematic review. Thyroid. 2010;**20**:1129-1138

[33] Fagin JA, Wells SA Jr. Biologic and clinical perspectives on thyroid cancer. The New England Journal of Medicine. 2016;**375**:1054-1067

[34] Cancer Genome Atlas Research Network. Integrated genomic characterization of papillary thyroid carcinoma. Cell. 2014;**159**:676-690

[35] Xing M, Westra WH, Tufano RP, Cohen Y, Rosenbaum E, Rhoden KJ, et al. BRAF mutation predicts a poorer clinical prognosis for papillary thyroid cancer. The Journal of Clinical Endocrinology and Metabolism. 2005;**90**:6373-6379

[36] Sabra MM, Dominguez JM, Grewal RK, Larson SM, Ghossein RA, Tuttle RM, et al. Clinical outcomes and molecular profile of differentiated thyroid cancers with radioiodine-avid distant metastases. The Journal of Clinical Endocrinology and Metabolism. 2013;**98**:E829-E836

[37] Xing M. Genetic-guided risk assessment and management of thyroid cancer. Endocrinology and Metabolism Clinics of North America. 2019;**48**:109-124

[38] Liu J, Liu R, Shen X, Zhu G, Li B, Xing M. The genetic duet of BRAF V600E and TERT promoter mutations robustly predicts loss of radioiodine avidity in recurrent papillary thyroid cancer. Journal of Nuclear Medicine. 2020;**61**:177-182

[39] Yang X, Li J, Li X, Liang Z, Gao W, Liang J, et al. TERT promoter mutation predicts radioiodine-refractory character in distant metastatic differentiated thyroid cancer. Journal of Nuclear Medicine. 2017;**58**:258-265

[40] Boucai L, Seshan V, Williams M, Knauf JA, Saqcena M, Ghossein RA, et al. Characterization of subtypes of BRAF-mutant papillary thyroid cancer defined by their thyroid differentiation score. The Journal of Clinical Endocrinology and Metabolism. 2022;**107**:1030-1039

[41] Seidlin SM, Marinelli LD, Oshry E. Radioactive iodine therapy; effect on functioning metastases of adenocarcinoma of the thyroid. Journal of the American Medical Association. 1946;**132**:838-847

[42] Schlumberger M, Brose M, Elisei R, Leboulleux S, Luster M, Pitoia F, et al. Definition and management of radioactive iodine-refractory differentiated thyroid cancer. The Lancet Diabetes and Endocrinology. 2014;**2**:356-358

[43] Kazahaya K, Prickett KK, Paulson VA, Dahl JP, Manning SC, Rudzinski ER, et al. Targeted oncogene therapy before surgery in pediatric patients with advanced invasive thyroid cancer at initial presentation: Is it time for a paradigm shift? JAMA Otolaryngology. Head & Neck Surgery. 2020;**146**:748-753

[44] Brose MS, Nutting CM, Jarzab B, Elisei R, Siena S, Bastholt L, et al. Sorafenib in radioactive iodine-refractory, locally advanced or metastatic differentiated thyroid cancer: A randomised, double-blind, phase 3 trial. Lancet. 2014;**384**:319-328

[45] Brose MS, Worden FP, Newbold KL, Guo M, Hurria A. Effect of age on the efficacy and safety of lenvatinib in radioiodine-refractory differentiated thyroid cancer in the Phase III SELECT Trial. Journal of Clinical Oncology. 2017;**35**:2692-2699

[46] Wirth LJ, Sherman E, Robinson B, Solomon B, Kang H, Lorch J, et al. Efficacy of selpercatinib in RET-altered thyroid cancers. The New England Journal of Medicine. 2020;**383**:825-835

[47] Drilon A, Laetsch TW, Kummar S, DuBois SG, Lassen UN, Demetri GD, et al. Efficacy of larotrectinib in TRK fusion-positive cancers in adults and children. The New England Journal of Medicine. 2018;**378**:731-739

[48] Riesco-Eizaguirre G, Santisteban P, De la Vieja A. The complex regulation of NIS expression and activity in thyroid and extrathyroidal tissues. Endocrine-Related Cancer. 2021;**28**:T141-T165

[49] Cazarin J, Dupuy C, Pires de Carvalho D. Redox homeostasis in thyroid cancer: Implications in Na(+)/I(-) symporter (NIS) regulation. International Journal of Molecular Sciences. 2022;**23**:6129

[50] Tavares C, Coelho MJ, Eloy C, Melo M, da Rocha AG, Pestana A, et al. NIS expression in thyroid tumors, relation with prognosis clinicopathological and molecular features. Endocrine Connections. 2018;**7**:78-90

[51] Dohan O, Baloch Z, Banrevi Z, Livolsi V, Carrasco N. Predominant intracellular overexpression of the Na(+)/I(-) symporter (NIS) in a large sampling of thyroid cancer cases. The Journal of Clinical Endocrinology and Metabolism. 2001;**86**:2697-2700

[52] Wapnir IL, van de Rijn M, Nowels K, Amenta PS, Walton K, Montgomery K, et al. Immunohistochemical profile of the sodium/iodide symporter in thyroid, breast, and other carcinomas using high density tissue microarrays and conventional sections. The Journal of Clinical Endocrinology and Metabolism. 2003;**88**:1880-1888

[53] Russo D, Manole D, Arturi F, Suarez HG, Schlumberger M,

Filetti S, et al. Absence of sodium/iodide symporter gene mutations in differentiated human thyroid carcinomas. Thyroid. 2001;**11**:37-39

[54] Neumann S, Schuchardt K, Reske A, Reske A, Emmrich P, Paschke R. Lack of correlation for sodium iodide symporter mRNA and protein expression and analysis of sodium iodide symporter promoter methylation in benign cold thyroid nodules. Thyroid. 2004;**14**:99-111

[55] Smith VE, Read ML, Turnell AS, Watkins RJ, Watkinson JC, Lewy GD, et al. A novel mechanism of sodium iodide symporter repression in differentiated thyroid cancer. Journal of Cell Science. 2009;**122**:3393-3402

[56] Smith VE, Sharma N, Watkins RJ, Read ML, Ryan GA, Kwan PP, et al. Manipulation of PBF/PTTG1IP phosphorylation status; a potential new therapeutic strategy for improving radioiodine uptake in thyroid tumors. The Journal of Clinical Endocrinology and Metabolism. 2013;**98**:2876-2886

[57] Fletcher A, Read ML, Thornton CEM, Larner DP, Poole VL, Brookes K, et al. Targeting novel sodium iodide symporter interactors ADP-ribosylation factor 4 and valosin-containing protein enhances radioiodine uptake. Cancer Research. 2020;**80**:102-115

[58] Read ML, Brookes K, Thornton CEM, Fletcher A, Nieto HR, Alshahrani M, et al. Targeting non-canonical pathways as a strategy to modulate the sodium iodide symporter. Cell Chemistry & Biology. 2022;**29**:502-516

[59] Amit M, Na'ara S, Francis D, Matanis W, Zolotov S, Eisenhaber B, et al. Post-translational regulation of radioactive iodine therapy response in papillary thyroid carcinoma. Journal of the National Cancer Institute. 2017;**109**:djx092

[60] Mitsutake N, Knauf JA, Mitsutake S, Mesa C Jr, Zhang L, Fagin JA. Conditional BRAFV600E expression induces DNA synthesis, apoptosis, dedifferentiation, and chromosomal instability in thyroid PCCL3 cells. Cancer Research. 2005;**65**:2465-2473

[61] Riesco-Eizaguirre G, Gutierrez-Martinez P, Garcia-Cabezas MA, Nistal M, Santisteban P. The oncogene BRAF V600E is associated with a high risk of recurrence and less differentiated papillary thyroid carcinoma due to the impairment of Na+/I- targeting to the membrane. Endocrine-Related Cancer. 2006;**13**:257-269

[62] Chakravarty D, Santos E, Ryder M, Knauf JA, Liao XH, West BL, et al. Small-molecule MAPK inhibitors restore radioiodine incorporation in mouse thyroid cancers with conditional BRAF activation. The Journal of Clinical Investigation. 2011;**121**:4700-4711

[63] Montero-Conde C, Ruiz-Llorente S, Dominguez JM, Knauf JA, Viale A, Sherman EJ, et al. Relief of feedback inhibition of HER3 transcription by RAF and MEK inhibitors attenuates their antitumor effects in BRAF-mutant thyroid carcinomas. Cancer Discovery. 2013;**3**:520-533

[64] Nagarajah J, Le M, Knauf JA, Ferrandino G, Montero-Conde C, Pillarsetty N, et al. Sustained ERK inhibition maximizes responses of BrafV600E thyroid cancers to radioiodine. The Journal of Clinical Investigation. 2016;**126**:4119-4124

[65] Lamartina L, Anizan N, Dupuy C, Leboulleux S, Schlumberger M. Redifferentiation-facilitated radioiodine therapy in thyroid

cancer. Endocrine-Related Cancer. 2021;**28**:T179-T191

[66] Ho AL, Grewal RK, Leboeuf R, Sherman EJ, Pfister DG, Deandreis D, et al. Selumetinib-enhanced radioiodine uptake in advanced thyroid cancer. The New England Journal of Medicine. 2013;**368**:623-632

[67] Rothenberg SM, McFadden DG, Palmer EL, Daniels GH, Wirth LJ. Redifferentiation of iodine-refractory BRAF V600E-mutant metastatic papillary thyroid cancer with dabrafenib. Clinical Cancer Research. 2015;**21**:1028-1035

[68] Dunn LA, Sherman EJ, Baxi SS, Tchekmedyian V, Grewal RK, Larson SM, et al. Vemurafenib redifferentiation of BRAF mutant, RAI-refractory thyroid cancers. The Journal of Clinical Endocrinology and Metabolism. 2019;**104**:1417-1428

[69] Iravani A, Solomon B, Pattison DA, Jackson P, Ravi Kumar A, Kong G, et al. Mitogen-activated protein kinase pathway inhibition for redifferentiation of radioiodine refractory differentiated thyroid cancer: An evolving protocol. Thyroid. 2019;**29**:1634-1645

[70] Ho AL, Dedecjus M, Wirth LJ, Tuttle RM, Inabnet WB 3rd, Tennvall J, et al. Selumetinib plus adjuvant radioactive iodine in patients with high-risk differentiated thyroid cancer: A Phase III, Randomized, Placebo-Controlled Trial (ASTRA). Journal of Clinical Oncology. 2022;**40**:1870-1878

[71] Cheng L, Jin Y, Liu M, Ruan M, Chen L. HER inhibitor promotes BRAF/MEK inhibitor-induced redifferentiation in papillary thyroid cancer harboring BRAFV600E. Oncotarget. 2017;**8**:19843-19854

[72] Tchekmedyian V, Dunn L, Sherman E, Baxi SS, Grewal RK, Larson SM, et al. Enhancing radioiodine incorporation in BRAF-mutant, radioiodine-refractory thyroid cancers with vemurafenib and the Anti-ErbB3 Monoclonal Antibody CDX-3379: Results of a Pilot Clinical Trial. Thyroid. 2022;**32**:273-282

[73] SaqcenaM,Leandro-GarciaLJ,MaagJLV, Tchekmedyian V, Krishnamoorthy GP, Tamarapu PP, et al. SWI/SNF complex mutations promote thyroid tumor progression and insensitivity to redifferentiation therapies. Cancer Discovery. 2021;**11**:1158-1175

[74] Groussin L, Theodon H, Bessiene L, Bricaire L, Bonnet-Serrano F, Cochand-Priollet B, et al. Redifferentiating effect of larotrectinib in NTRK-rearranged advanced radioactive-iodine refractory thyroid cancer. Thyroid. 2022;**32**:594-598

[75] Lee YA, Lee H, Im SW, Song YS, Oh DY, Kang HJ, et al. NTRK and RET fusion-directed therapy in pediatric thyroid cancer yields a tumor response and radioiodine uptake. The Journal of Clinical Investigation. 2021;**131**:e144847

[76] Groussin L, Clerc J, Huillard O. Larotrectinib-enhanced radioactive iodine uptake in advanced thyroid cancer. The New England Journal of Medicine. 2020;**383**:1686-1687

[77] Groussin L, Bessiene L, Arrondeau J, Garinet S, Cochand-Priollet B, Lupo A, et al. Letter to the editor: Selpercatinib-enhanced radioiodine uptake in RET-rearranged thyroid cancer. Thyroid. 2021;**31**:1603-1604

[78] Waguespack SG, Tewari SO, Busaidy NL, Zafereo ME. Larotrectinib before initial radioactive iodine therapy in pediatric TRK fusion-positive

papillary thyroid carcinoma: Time to reconsider the treatment paradigm for distantly metastatic disease? JCO Precision Oncology. 2022;**6**:e2100467

[79] Maxon HR, Thomas SR, Hertzberg VS, Kereiakes JG, Chen IW, Sperling MI, et al. Relation between effective radiation dose and outcome of radioiodine therapy for thyroid cancer. The New England Journal of Medicine. 1983;**309**:937-941

[80] Lakshmanan A, Scarberry D, Green JA, Zhang X, Selmi-Ruby S, Jhiang SM. Modulation of thyroidal radioiodide uptake by oncological pipeline inhibitors and Apigenin. Oncotarget. 2015;**6**:31792-31804

Section 2

Treatment of Thyroid Cancer

Chapter 5

Thyroid Cancer: From Genes to Treatment – Recent Developments

Ifigenia Kostoglou-Athanassiou

Abstract

Thyroid cancer carries a good prognosis in most cases and is treated by thyroidectomy, radioiodine administration thereafter, thyroxine treatment. Although, most cases of thyroid cancer are curable, if thyroid cancer loses the ability to concentrate iodine and thus becomes refractory to radioiodine, and if thyroid cancer becomes a progressive disease, the need for targeted treatment becomes necessary. Research in the area of the biology of thyroid cancer and in particular the discovery of somatic genetic mutations involved in the pathophysiology of thyroid cancer as well as research in the treatment of other cancer types with tyrosine kinase inhibitors have led to the application of tyrosine kinase and angiogenetic factor inhibitors in the treatment of thyroid cancer. The application of tyrosine kinase inhibitors in other tumor types led to the discovery that they target the thyroid. Thus, tyrosine kinase inhibitors entered the field of radioactive iodine refractory and advanced thyroid cancer treatment. Multi-kinase and angiogenetic factor inhibitors have provided a novel method that targets thyroid tumors and have revolutionized the treatment of radioiodine refractory and advanced thyroid cancer.

Keywords: tyrosine kinase inhibitors, multi-kinase and angiogenetic factor inhibitors, advanced thyroid cancer, iodine refractory thyroid cancer, differentiated thyroid cancer, medullary thyroid carcinoma

1. Introduction

Thyroid cancer represents 90% of malignant tumors of the endocrine system and is the cause of 0.5% of all deaths from cancer in man [1–3]. Thyroid cancer is quite frequent, as in adults in autopsy findings it has been observed with a frequency ranging from 4 to 36% [4]. In the clinical setting, thyroid cancer is found in 6–10% of thyroid nodules [5]. Thyroid cancer is observed with greater prevalence in female as compared to male patients with a rate of 2–3/1 [6]. The incidence of thyroid cancer was rising until recently in the USA; however, its incidence now has leveled off. The main types of thyroid cancer are the two types of differentiated follicular thyroid carcinoma, namely papillary and follicular, representing 70–80% and 15–20%, respectively, and medullary and anaplastic thyroid carcinomas with a frequency of 5–8% and 3–5%, respectively (**Figure 1**) [7]. The etiology of thyroid cancer includes genetic mutations, head and neck irradiation, and iodine deficiency [8]. The diagnosis is

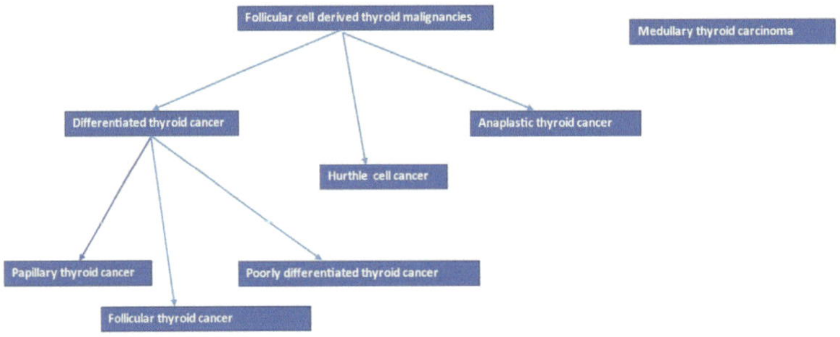

Figure 1.
Histological types of thyroid cancer.

based on history, clinical examination, biochemical and imaging examination, and fine needle aspiration biopsy [9]. Treatment of differentiated and medullary thyroid carcinoma is total or near total thyroidectomy, including lymph node dissection [10, 11]. In differentiated thyroid carcinoma, radioactive iodine is administered for the destruction of thyroid remnants [12]. In anaplastic thyroid carcinoma, an effort is made for resection of as much as possible of the tumor. In all cases, thyroxine treatment is administered [13]. The prognosis of differentiated thyroid cancer is good and 10-year prognosis in papillary thyroid cancer is 93%, in follicular thyroid cancer is 85%, in medullary thyroid cancer 75%, and in anaplastic thyroid cancer 2–6 months, while rarely more than a year [14].

Although, most cases of thyroid cancer are curable, if thyroid cancer loses the ability to concentrate iodine and thus becomes refractory to radioiodine and if thyroid cancer becomes a progressive disease the need for targeted treatment becomes necessary [15]. Novel treatment methods for the management of advanced thyroid cancer have emerged after extensive research efforts, which have revolutionized thyroid cancer treatment [16–22]. Research in the area of the biology of thyroid cancer and in particular the discovery of somatic genetic mutations [23, 24] involved in the pathophysiology of thyroid cancer as well as research in the treatment of other cancer types with tyrosine kinase inhibitors [25] have led to the application of tyrosine kinase and angiogenetic factor inhibitors in the treatment of thyroid cancer [26]. In cases of renal cancer, the application of tyrosine kinase inhibitors led to the appearance of hypothyroidism due to the destruction of the thyroid gland [27, 28]. Thus, tyrosine kinase entered the field of radioactive iodine refractory and advanced thyroid cancer [29]. Multi-kinase and angiogenetic factor inhibitors have revolutionized the treatment of radioiodine refractory and advanced thyroid cancer [29]. The need for genetic mutation testing before treatment is initiated [30, 31] has been recognized in patients with radioiodine refractory and advanced thyroid cancer to enable targeted treatment.

2. Molecular genetics in the etiology of thyroid cancer

The etiology of thyroid cancer is not known, although there are factors known to induce its development, such as ionizing radiation and iodine deficiency. Recent progress in molecular genetics has shown that thyroid cancer is due to genetic mutations either germline or somatic (**Figure 2**) [32]. These mutations lead to the inactivation of

DOI: http://dx.doi.org/10.5772/intechopen.111701

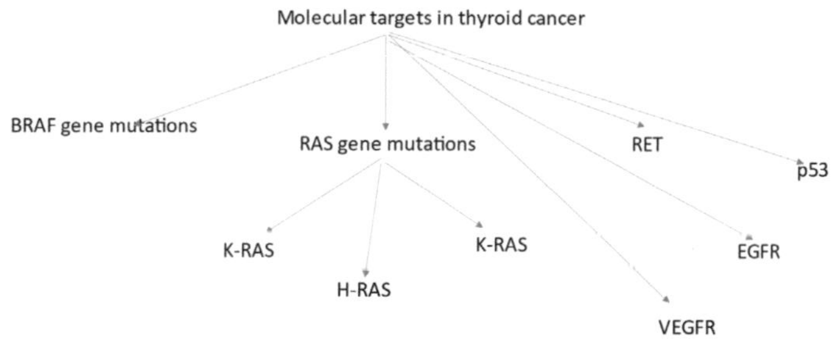

Figure 2.
Molecular targets in thyroid cancer.

onco-suppressor genes, which inhibit the formation of cancer or to the activation of oncogenes, which act on normal cells and lead to cancer development.

Papillary thyroid carcinoma is the most common thyroid cancer and represents approximately 80% of cases. Papillary thyroid carcinomas frequently harbor genetic changes leading to the activation of the mitogen-activated protein kinase (MAPK) signaling pathway [33]. These genetic alterations are mainly the RET/PTC rearrangement and point mutations of the BRAF and RAS genes. Mutations involving the above-mentioned genes are observed in more than 70% of papillary carcinomas and are mutually exclusive, meaning that if one mutation is found the other is not observed [32]. Genetic changes observed in follicular carcinomas, which represent the second in frequency type of thyroid cancer, are RAS mutations and PAX8-PPARγ rearrangement [33]. The discovery of these mutations led to extensive research and the discovery of therapeutic agents for the successful management of iodine refractory or advanced thyroid cancer.

In papillary thyroid cancer, the most common genetic mutation which has been observed is the gene rearrangement of the RET gene, which leads to increased expression of tyrosine kinase [34]. Thus, the thyroid cell is led to increased growth and multiplication and finally to tumor formation.

Follicular thyroid cancer presents with mutations in RAS oncogenes, which cause cell growth and multiplication [33]. The presence of RAS mutations is also observed in papillary carcinomas with follicular differentiation. Ionizing radiation is a known etiologic factor for thyroid cancer. It appears that small energy sources are transferred with radiation to the cells, leading subsequently to RAS gene mutations.

Anaplastic thyroid carcinoma has mutations in p53 gene [35, 36]. The p53 gene is a translational factor that is involved in the regulation of apoptosis and the cell cycle. It appears that this is the final step in the formation of thyroid cancer with the most malignant phenotype, which is added to the already existing genetic changes.

Medullary thyroid cancer presents with mutations in RET oncogene [37]. There has been progress in the pathogenesis of medullary thyroid carcinoma both in the hereditary and sporadic medullary thyroid carcinoma. The RET gene is involved in the pathogenesis of hereditary and sporadic medullary thyroid carcinoma. Mutations observed in the germ cells are detected in all the cells of the organism and their detection in the DNA of blood leucocytes forms the basis of finding carriers of the MEN2 syndrome. The MEN2 syndrome diagnosis is based on finding medullary thyroid cancer, pheochromocytoma, and parathyroid adenoma. In 97% of patients mutations in the RET gene have been observed in the DNA of blood leucocytes. In sporadic medullary thyroid carcinoma, somatic RET mutations at the level of the thyroid tumor have been observed.

3. Genetic mutations and thyroid cancer

3.1 BRAF

The most studied point mutation in thyroid cancer is that of the BRAF gene [33, 34]. The $BRAF^{v600E}$ somatic mutation is involved in approximately 45% of papillary thyroid cancer and tall cell variant and in 25% of anaplastic thyroid cancer. This somatic mutation of thyroid cells is related to the substitution of valine with glutamate and leads to the activation of BRAF kinase, which phosphorylates several targets and in particular mitogen-activated protein kinase (MEK) and extracellular signal-regulated kinase (ERK) [38]. The $BRAF^{v600E}$ mutation is associated with tumor aggressiveness and a poor prognosis, as it leads to higher tumor size and metastasis, either lymph node or distant metastasis.

3.2 RET/PTC

The RET proto-oncogene codes for a cell membrane receptor tyrosine kinase. Within the thyroid, RET is expressed in parafollicular C cells, within which it can be activated by chromosomal rearrangement. In RET/PTC the 3′ portion of the RET gene is fused to the 5′ portion of various unrelated genes [39]. The RET/PTC1 and RET/PTC3 account for most of the rearrangements observed in papillary carcinomas. RET/PTC is tumorigenic in thyroid follicular cells and is detected in approximately 20% of papillary thyroid carcinomas. Papillary thyroid carcinomas with RET/PTC rearrangement present at a younger age, have lymph node metastases and may have a favorable prognosis.

3.3 RAS

Another frequent driver of somatic mutation involved in the pathogenesis of thyroid cancer is that of the RAS gene [40], which lies upstream of BRAF. N-RAS, H-RAS, and K-RAS are members of the RAS family and those most commonly involved in thyroid cancer are the N-RAS and H-RAS and can constitutively activate the MAPK and PI3K/AKT pathways. RAS somatic mutations are present in 40–50% of follicular thyroid cancer, 15% of papillary thyroid cancer, follicular variant thyroid cancer, and 50% of anaplastic thyroid cancer. The K-RAS mutation is considered an activator of the MAPK pathway as compared to N-RAS mutation, which is an activator of the PI3K-AKT pathway. In papillary thyroid cancer genetic mutations of the RAS gene are mutually exclusive with the mutations of the BRAF gene.

3.4 RET point mutations

In medullary thyroid carcinomas, RET is activated by point mutations, as compared to its activation by chromosomal rearrangement in papillary thyroid cancer. Germline mutations are observed in MEN2A, MEN2B, and familial medullary thyroid

DOI: http://dx.doi.org/10.5772/intechopen.111701

carcinoma [41]. In MEN2A most mutations affect codon 634, whereas in MEN2B germline mutations affect codon 918, whereas in sporadic medullary thyroid carcinomas, somatic mutations of RET are observed [42].

3.5 VEGF

Angiogenesis has a key role in tumor initiation and progression and lymphangio genesis is crucial for metastasis formation. Thus, angiogenesis and lymphangiogenesis are targets of cancer treatment. Angiogenesis involves the activation of VEGFR2, a tyrosine kinase receptor that is expressed in vascular endothelial cells. The expression of VEGFR2, a tyrosine kinase receptor is induced by VEGF-A produced by neoplastic and immune cells within the tumor.

Hypoxia within the tumor induces the activation of transcriptional factor hypoxia-inducible factor-1 alpha (HIF-1α), which leads to expression of VEGF-A. HIF-1α is expressed mainly in anaplastic thyroid cancer cells.

Thyroid cancer aggressiveness is associated with increased angiogenesis and the expression of VEGF/VEGFR, PDGF/PDGFR, and EGF/EGFR [43, 44]. In differentiated thyroid cancer, VEGFR and VEGFR-2 are overexpressed and contribute to tumor progression and aggressiveness. In particular, in papillary thyroid cancer, VEGF expression is related to local and distant metastatic disease.

3.6 EGFR

The EGFR cell surface protein is a member of the ErbB family of receptors. In epithelial carcinoma, EGFR mutations have been observed. EGFR has been found to be related to thyroid cancer progression and invasiveness and its overexpression has been observed in anaplastic thyroid cancer [45].

3.7 Tumor suppressor genes

The gene tumor protein P53 (TP53) encodes the tumor suppressor gene p53. The loss of its expression leads to a loss of control of cell growth and cell apoptosis. The p53 gene is mutated in anaplastic thyroid cancer and is involved in its pathogenesis [35, 46].

4. Multi-kinase and angiogenetic factor inhibitors

The successful application of multi-kinase and angiogenetic factor inhibitors in the treatment of various types of cancer [25] has led to observations that multiple kinase and angiogenetic factor inhibitors attack the thyroid cells and may lead to hypothyroidism and in some cases eradication of the thyroid gland [27, 28, 47]. These observations led to the application of multi-kinase and angiogenetic factor inhibitors in the treatment of radioactive iodine refractory and advanced thyroid cancer (**Table 1**) [37]. Multi-kinase and angiogenetic factor inhibitors interfere with some of the pathogenetic pathways involved in the pathogenesis of thyroid cancer and in tumor growth and the development of metastatic disease [10]. This application has led to a revolution in the treatment of advanced thyroid cancer.

Drug	Target—mode of action	Indications by histology of thyroid cancer
Axitinib	TKI VEGFR1–3	DTC, MTC, ATC
Cabozantinib	TKI, VEGFR2, MET, FLT3, RET, c-kit	MTC, DTC
Dabrafenib	STKI, $BRAF^{V600E}$	DTC
Dabrafenib with trametinib	STKI, $BRAF^{V600E}$, MEK1/2	DTC
Entrectinib	TrkI, NTRK fusions	DTC
Larotrectinib	TrkI, NTRK fusions	NTRK-fusion thyroid carcinoma
Pazopanib	TKI, VEGFR1–3 PDGFR, FGFR1/2, c-kit	MTC, DTC, ATC
Sorafenib	TKI, VEGFR1–3, PDGFR, RET, c-kit, CSF-1R, Flt-3	DTC, MTC, ATC
Sunitinib	TKI: VEGFR1–3, PDGFR, RET, c-kit, CSF-1R, Flt-3	MTC
Vandetanib	TKI, VEGFR2/3, EGFR, RET	MTC, DTC
Vemurafenib	STKI, $BRAF^{V600E}$	DTC

TKI—tyrosine kinase inhibitor, STKI—serine-threonine kinase inhibitor, DTC—differentiated thyroid cancer, MTC—medullary thyroid cancer, ATC—anaplastic thyroid cancer.

Table 1.
Drugs applied in the treatment of advanced thyroid cancer.

4.1 Sunitinib

Sunitinib is a small molecule and is a multi-kinase and angiogenetic factor inhibitor that inhibits RET/PTC subtypes 1 and 3, VEGFR1, VEGFR-2, VGEFR-3, KIT, and PDGFR kinases [48]. The drug was initially approved by the FDA for gastrointestinal stromal tumor and clear cell renal carcinoma [49]. The drug is currently under investigation for the treatment of several human tumors. The most common adverse events are hand-foot syndrome, fatigue, neutropenia, diarrhea, hypothyroidism, and hypertension [50].

Sunitinib was found in preclinical studies to inhibit *in vitro* RET/PTC oncoproteins. It has been studied in various studies in differentiated thyroid cancer and medullary thyroid cancer patients and either partial response or stable disease was observed [51, 52]. In a study with metastatic radioiodine-refractory thyroid cancer partial response was observed. In the phase II trial of sunitinib (THYSU), the drug was tested in patients with advanced or metastatic differentiated/anaplastic or medullary thyroid cancer with improvement in progression-free survival and overall survival [53, 54]. In the phase II trial of sunitinib in progressive medullary thyroid cancer patients, the drug was found to be effective in progressive medullary thyroid cancer. In an open-label phase II study, sunitinib was found to induce complete response in some patients with metastatic medullary thyroid cancer and differentiated thyroid cancer. In an anaplastic thyroid cancer patient, sunitinib was administered with a good clinical response [55].

4.2 Sorafenib

Sorafenib is a multi-kinase inhibitor that inhibits RAF, VEGFR2, VEGFR3, PDGFR, RET, and KIT kinases [56, 57]. It exerts anti-neoplasmatic effects in preclinical models of cancer and thyroid cancer cell lines. Sorafenib inhibits thyroid cancer growth by acting with antiproliferative and antiangiogenic mechanisms [57]. The FDA has approved its use in hepatocellular and renal cell carcinoma and metastatic differentiated thyroid carcinoma [58]. Sorafenib is administered orally at 400 mg twice daily and is usually well tolerated. Sorafenib has been administered to patients with metastatic radioiodine refractory thyroid cancer for about 27 weeks and it was found to induce a partial response, improve progression-free survival and have clinical benefits [59]. In another study, sorafenib was administered to patients with metastatic papillary thyroid cancer chemotherapy-naive and in patients with papillary thyroid cancer who had already received chemotherapy and other subtypes of thyroid cancer and it was found to induce partial response in 6 of 22 patients and to induce disease stabilization which lasted more than 6 months in 23 patients [59, 60]. Sorafenib was administered to radioactive iodine refractory papillary and follicular thyroid cancer with a remission rate of 20% [59]. In these patients with metastatic thyroid cancer, the response of metastatic disease differed depending on the site of metastasis. Bone lesions had a minimal response, whereas a better effect was observed in lung metastatic disease. Thyroglobulin was considered a positive biomarker of response to treatment. In a double-blind phase III trial, the clinical activity of sorafenib as compared to placebo was assessed in patients with radioactive iodine refractory locally advanced or metastatic differentiated thyroid carcinoma [17]. In patients treated with sorafenib, the progress-free survival increased in all subgroups regardless of mutation status. This study demonstrated the efficacy of sorafenib in radioactive–iodine refractory differentiated thyroid cancer. Other studies demonstrated the efficacy of sorafenib in progressive metastatic differentiated thyroid cancer. A meta-analysis involving 15 studies evaluated the safety and efficacy of sorafenib in radioactive iodine refractory differentiated thyroid carcinoma [59]. Sorafenib improved progression-free survival in patients with radioactive iodine refractory differentiated thyroid carcinoma patients. The most frequent adverse effects were hand-foot syndrome, diarrhea, fatigue, alopecia, weight loss, and rash. The study focused on the efficacy of sorafenib in improving progression-free survival in differentiated thyroid cancer as compared to placebo. Although sorafenib was observed in combination with metformin to inhibit anaplastic thyroid cancer cells [61], the drug was not effective *in vivo* in an anaplastic thyroid cancer patient [36].

Sorafenib is associated with an increase in progression-free survival and disease stabilization. Sorafenib administration and acquired resistance to it may be associated with the induction of autophagy [62]. In this context, several substances have been applied to limit autophagy and the related resistance of cancer to treatment [62, 63]. The administration of agents to inhibit autophagy may sensitize a tumor to the multi-kinase inhibitor linifanib [64].

4.3 Vandetanib

Vandetanib is a potent inhibitor of VEGFR-2, VEGFR-3, RET, and EGFR kinases [65]. Vandetanib has been approved by FDA and EMA for use in patients with metastatic or progressive medullary thyroid cancer [66]. In an international randomized trial, the therapeutic efficacy of vandetanib was shown in patients with advanced medullary thyroid cancer as it showed a significant prolongation of progression-free survival as compared to placebo [67]. In a double-blind phase II study, vandetanib was shown to prolong progression-free survival in patients with locally advanced or metastatic differentiated thyroid carcinoma patients [68]. Recently, a meta-analysis and systematic review, through standardized RECIST criteria as endpoints, investigated vandetanib efficacy in medullary thyroid carcinoma. The study included only original studies in which the drug was used as a single agent. Ten (eight observational longitudinal studies and two randomized controlled trials) were included among the 487 screened articles. The results obtained through the RECIST criteria did not provide clear evidence of the efficacy of vandetanib [69]. Nonetheless, vandetanib is considered a new-generation treatment in advanced medullary thyroid carcinoma.

Vandetanib has been evaluated in patients with symptomatic or progressive medullary thyroid cancer in various starting doses, 150 or 300 mg daily, and was found to have a good response with a better response at the dose of 300 mg [70]. Adverse effects of vandetanib were QTc prolongation, hypocalcemia, asthenia, diarrhea, keratopathy, and hypokalemia. In a systematic review, the cost-effectiveness of cabozantinib and vandetanib were compared [71]. Both drugs improved progress-free survival although no significant overall survival benefits were observed. Vandetanib is considered a new-generation treatment for advanced medullary thyroid cancer.

4.4 Lenvatinib

Lenvatinib inhibits FGFR-1, FGFR-2, FGFR-3, FGFR-4, PGGFRβ, VEGFR-1, VEGFR-2, VEGFR-3, RET, and KIT kinases [72]. Lenvatinib has been approved by FDA and EMA for the treatment of advanced radioactive iodine refractory differentiated thyroid cancer [73]. Lenvatinib was administered to patients with advanced radioiodine refractory differentiated thyroid cancer that had progressed during the earlier 12 months. After a follow-up of 14 months, the overall response rate was 50%, the median time to relapse was 3.6 months, the median progression-free survival was 12.6 months and the median response duration was 12.7 months. Lenvatinib was administered to patients with unresectable progressive medullary thyroid cancer and was found to be effective [74]. In a double-blind randomized study, lenvatinib was administered to 261 patients with progressive radioiodine refractory thyroid carcinoma [16]. The study included a placebo group of 131 patients. Median progression-free survival was longer in the lenvatinib group as compared to placebo. The response rate was 64.8%. However, side effects were observed. In a randomized study examining the effect of lenvatinib on tumor size, it was shown to improve tumor size rapidly at the beginning of the study and to induce continued shrinkage thereafter [75]. A phase II study evaluated lenvatinib in 51 patients with radioactive iodine refractory differentiated thyroid carcinoma, medullary thyroid carcinoma, and anaplastic thyroid cancer with a median progression-free survival of 25.8 months, 9.2 months, and 7.4 months, respectively [76]. The safety profile of the drug was manageable, and an antitumor efficacy was observed in radioactive iodine refractory thyroid cancer and promising efficacy in medullary thyroid cancer and anaplastic thyroid cancer. Lenvatinib was also evaluated postoperatively in anaplastic thyroid cancer patients and was shown to have a response rate of 17.4% [77]. Hypertension was the most frequent adverse effect.

4.5 Cabozantinib

Cabozantinib inhibits Tie-2, c-MET, KIT, VEGFR-1, VEGFR-2, and RET kinases [78]. In a phase I trial, cabozantinib was administered to patients with advanced solid tumors, including 37 patients with advanced medullary thyroid cancer, and was found to have efficacy and a good safety profile in medullary thyroid cancer as it induced tumor shrinkage of >30% in some medullary thyroid cancer patients with measurable disease [79]. Cabozantinib was also evaluated in 15 radioiodine refractory differentiated thyroid cancer patients who had progressed on conventional treatment and had measurable disease [80]. FDA-approved cabozantinib for the treatment of metastatic medullary thyroid cancer. Cabozantinib was also evaluated in patients with advanced radioiodine refractory differentiated thyroid cancer who had already received another VEGFR-targeted treatment and was found to be clinically effective [81]. In a double-blind phase III trial, cabozantinib was found to be effective in improving progression-free survival in patients with progressive medullary thyroid cancer [82].

4.6 Dabrafenib and trametinib

Dabrafenib (also known as GSK2118436) is a BRAF kinase inhibitor, which has been tested *in vitro* and has demonstrated antiproliferative effects in human colon cancer xenografts and $BRAF^{V600E}$ positive melanoma [83]. It has also been tested in clinical trials in BRAF-positive cancers. In this case, BRAF-positive cancers become resistant to dabrafenib in 6–7 months. To prevent this therapeutic failure dabrafenib was administered with trametinib, a MEK inhibitor, and this combination was approved by the FDA for the treatment of $BRAF^{V600E}$ positive metastatic melanoma. Dabrafenib and trametinib were administered to anaplastic cancer patients with $BRAF^{V600E}$ mutation with promising results [55, 84–87].

4.7 Pazopanib

Pazopanib has been tested for advanced thyroid cancer and RET-mutant medullary thyroid cancer [88]. It can be used to treat advanced papillary or follicular thyroid cancer if they express RET gene changes. Pazopanib is an oral small-molecule multi-kinase inhibitor that primarily inhibits vascular endothelial growth factor receptor-1, -2, and -3, platelet endothelial growth factor receptor-α, and -β, and the stem-cell factor receptor c-kit [89]. Pazopanib was introduced as a treatment against various tumors and it has been approved in several countries for advanced soft-tissue sarcoma and renal cell carcinoma. Large clinical trials with pazopanib in patients having soft-tissue sarcoma and renal cell carcinoma have shown beneficial effects. Adverse events include liver dysfunction and hypertension but are generally manageable. Pazopanib has also been used in patients with advanced thyroid cancer [90].

4.8 Selpercatinib

Selpercatinib is a receptor tyrosine kinase RET (rearranged during transfection) inhibitor developed for the treatment of cancers harboring RET alterations [22]. Selpercatinib was approved by the FDA for the treatment of RET fusion-positive non-small cell lung cancer, RET fusion-positive thyroid.

4.9 Larotrectinib

Larotrectinib is a selective and specific inhibitor of tropomyosin receptor kinase A (TRKA), TRKB, and TRKC approved for use in Europe and the USA, which is used in the therapy of solid tumors harboring NTRK gene fusions. NTRK gene fusions involving either NTRK1, NTRK2, or NTRK3 (encoding the neurotrophin receptors TRKA, TRKB, and TRKC, respectively) are oncogenic drivers of various adult and pediatric tumor types. It has been applied in thyroid tumors thought to harbor NTRK gene fusions [91] and has been approved by the FDA for tumor agnostic indications.

4.10 Entrectinib

Entrectinib is another inhibitor of TRKA, TRKB, and TRKC. It has been applied in the treatment of NTRK fusion-positive cancers, including thyroid cancer [92]. Thyroid cancer-specific data are not yet available for entrectinib.

4.11 Vemurafenib

Vemurafenib was developed as a low-molecular-weight molecule for the inhibition of the mutated serine-threonine kinase BRAF, and it selectively binds to the ATP-binding site of $BRAF^{v600E}$ kinase and inhibits its activity [93]. It has potential to be applied in papillary thyroid carcinoma, which harbors a BRAF mutation.

5. Mutational testing in thyroid cancer

Most thyroid cancer cases carry a good prognosis. However, 15% of differentiated thyroid cancer cases present with locally advanced disease, and in radioiodine refractory thyroid cancer 10-year survival drops below 50%. Patients with advanced thyroid cancer and radioiodine refractory thyroid cancer should undergo somatic mutational screening [94], as novel drugs are available to treat them. These drugs are the novel multiple kinase and angiogenetic factor inhibitors, which have offered patients and physicians a new option for the treatment of advanced thyroid cancer and have revolutionized the treatment of advanced thyroid cancer patients.

6. Conclusion

The application of multi-kinase and angiogenetic factor inhibitors in the treatment of radioiodine refractory and advanced thyroid cancer has enabled the successful management of the disease and has revolutionized the management of radioiodine refractory and advanced thyroid cancer. As the application of these multi-kinase and angiogenetic factor inhibitors is related with an increase in progression-free survival and disease stabilization, further research is needed to identify the mechanisms involved in the acquired resistance to these agents and the ways to manage this resistance. Mutational testing in thyroid cancer may contribute to the application of targeted treatment.

Acknowledgements

The help of Professor Sylviane Muller, University of Strasbourg Institute for Advanced Study/Chair Therapeutic Immunology, in revising the chapter is gratefully acknowledged.

Author details

Ifigenia Kostoglou-Athanassiou
Department of Endocrinology, Asclepeion Hospital, Voula, Athens, Greece

*Address all correspondence to: ikostoglouathanassiou@yahoo.gr

References

[1] Cabanillas ME, McFadden DG, Durante C. Thyroid cancer. Lancet. 2016;**388**(10061):2783-2795. DOI: 10.1016/s0140-6736(16)30172-6

[2] Roman BR, Morris LG, Davies L. The thyroid cancer epidemic, 2017 perspective. Current Opinion in Endocrinology, Diabetes, and Obesity. 2017;**24**(5):332-336. DOI: 10.1097/med.0000000000000359

[3] Carling T, Udelsman R. Thyroid cancer. Annual Review of Medicine. 2014;**65**:125-137. DOI: 10.1146/annurev-med-061512-105739

[4] Dean DS, Gharib H. Epidemiology of thyroid nodules. Best Practice & Research. Clinical Endocrinology & Metabolism. 2008;**22**(6):901-911. DOI: 10.1016/j.beem.2008.09.019

[5] Grani G, Sponziello M, Pecce V, Ramundo V, Durante C. Contemporary thyroid nodule evaluation and management. The Journal of Clinical Endocrinology and Metabolism. 2020;**105**(9):2869-2883. DOI: 10.1210/clinem/dgaa322

[6] Suteau V, Munier M, Briet C, Rodien P. Sex bias in differentiated thyroid cancer. International Journal of Molecular Sciences. 2021;**22**:23. DOI: 10.3390/ijms222312992

[7] Clark OH, Duh QY. Thyroid cancer. The Medical Clinics of North America. 1991;**75**(1):211-234. DOI: 10.1016/s0025-7125(16)30480-1

[8] Yakushina VD, Lerner LV, Lavrov AV. Gene fusions in thyroid Cancer. Thyroid. 2018;**28**(2):158-167. DOI: 10.1089/thy.2017.0318

[9] Lincango-Naranjo E, Solis-Pazmino P, El Kawkgi O, et al. Triggers of thyroid cancer diagnosis: A systematic review and meta-analysis. Endocrine. 2021;**72**(3):644-659. DOI: 10.1007/s12020-020-02588-8

[10] Schmidbauer B, Menhart K, Hellwig D, Grosse J. Differentiated thyroid cancer-treatment: State of the art. International Journal of Molecular Science. 2017;**18**(6):1292. DOI: 10.3390/ijms18061292

[11] Araque KA, Gubbi S, Klubo-Gwiezdzinska J. Updates on the management of thyroid cancer. Hormone and Metabolic Research. 2020;**52**(8):562-577. DOI: 10.1055/a-1089-7870

[12] Ciarallo A, Rivera J. Radioactive iodine therapy in differentiated thyroid Cancer: 2020 update. AJR. American Journal of Roentgenology. 2020;**215**(2):285-291. DOI: 10.2214/ajr.19.22626

[13] Bible KC, Kebebew E, Brierley J, et al. 2021 American Thyroid Association Guidelines for management of patients with anaplastic thyroid cancer. Thyroid. 2021;**31**(3):337-386. DOI: 10.1089/thy.2020.0944

[14] Chmielik E, Rusinek D, Oczko-Wojciechowska M, et al. Heterogeneity of thyroid cancer. Pathobiology. 2018;**85**(1-2):117-129. DOI: 10.1159/000486422

[15] Haddad RI. New developments in thyroid cancer. Journal of the National Comprehensive Cancer Network. 2013;**11**(5 Suppl):705-707. DOI: 10.6004/jnccn.2013.0207

[16] Schlumberger M, Tahara M, Wirth LJ, et al. Lenvatinib versus placebo

in radioiodine-refractory thyroid cancer. New England Journal of Medicine. 2015;**372**(7):621-630. DOI: 10.1056/NEJMoa1406470

[17] Brose MS, Nutting CM, Jarzab B, et al. Sorafenib in radioactive iodine-refractory, locally advanced or metastatic differentiated thyroid cancer: A randomised, double-blind, phase 3 trial. Lancet. 2014;**384**(9940):319-328. DOI: 10.1016/s0140-6736(14)60421-9

[18] Haugen BR. American Thyroid Association management guidelines for adult patients with thyroid nodules and differentiated thyroid cancer: What is new and what has changed? Cancer. 2015, 2017;**123**(3):372-381. DOI: 10.1002/cncr.30360

[19] Jaber T, Waguespack SG, Cabanillas ME, et al. Targeted therapy in advanced thyroid cancer to Resensitize Tumors to radioactive iodine. The Journal of Clinical Endocrinology and Metabolism. 2018;**103**(10):3698-3705. DOI: 10.1210/jc.2018-00612

[20] Yeung KT, Cohen EE. Lenvatinib in advanced, radioactive iodine-refractory, differentiated thyroid carcinoma. Clinical Cancer Research. 2015;**21**(24):5420-5426. DOI: 10.1158/1078-0432.ccr-15-0923

[21] Capdevila J, Wirth LJ, Ernst T, et al. PD-1 blockade in anaplastic thyroid carcinoma. Journal of Clinical Oncology. 2020;**38**(23):2620-2627. DOI: 10.1200/jco.19.02727

[22] Wirth LJ, Sherman E, Robinson B, et al. Efficacy of Selpercatinib in RET-altered thyroid cancers. The New England Journal of Medicine. 2020;**383**(9):825-835. DOI: 10.1056/NEJMoa2005651

[23] Sherman SI, Clary DO, Elisei R, et al. Correlative analyses of RET and RAS mutations in a phase 3 trial of cabozantinib in patients with progressive, metastatic medullary thyroid cancer. Cancer. 2016;**122**(24):3856-3864. DOI: 10.1002/cncr.30252

[24] Nikiforova MN, Nikiforov YE. Molecular diagnostics and predictors in thyroid cancer. Thyroid. 2009;**19**(12):1351-1361. DOI: 10.1089/thy.2009.0240

[25] Rini BI, Pal SK, Escudier BJ, et al. Tivozanib versus sorafenib in patients with advanced renal cell carcinoma (TIVO-3): A phase 3, multicentre, randomised, controlled, open-label study. The Lancet Oncology. 2020;**21**(1):95-104. DOI: 10.1016/s1470-2045(19)30735-1

[26] Xing M, Haugen BR, Schlumberger M. Progress in molecular-based management of differentiated thyroid cancer. Lancet. 2013;**381**(9871):1058-1069. DOI: 10.1016/s0140-6736(13)60109-9

[27] Sabatier R, Eymard JC, Walz J, et al. Could thyroid dysfunction influence outcome in sunitinib-treated metastatic renal cell carcinoma? Annals of Oncology. 2012;**23**(3):714-721. DOI: 10.1093/annonc/mdr275

[28] Kitajima K, Takahashi S, Maeda T, et al. Thyroid size change by CT monitoring after sorafenib or sunitinib treatment in patients with renal cell carcinoma: Comparison with thyroid function. European Journal of Radiology. 2012;**81**(9):2060-2065. DOI: 10.1016/j.ejrad.2011.06.035

[29] Fagin JA, Tuttle RM, Pfister DG. Harvesting the low-hanging fruit: Kinase inhibitors for therapy of advanced medullary and nonmedullary thyroid cancer. The Journal of Clinical

Endocrinology and Metabolism. 2010;**6**:2621-2624

[30] Laha D, Nilubol N, Boufraqech M. New therapies for advanced thyroid cancer. Frontiers in Endocrinology (Lausanne). 2020;**11**:82. DOI: 10.3389/fendo.2020.00082

[31] Roth MY, Witt RL, Steward DL. Molecular testing for thyroid nodules: Review and current state. Cancer. 2018;**124**(5):888-898. DOI: 10.1002/cncr.30708

[32] Soares P, Trovisco V, Rocha AS, et al. BRAF mutations and RET/PTC rearrangements are alternative events in the etiopathogenesis of PTC. Oncogene. 2003;**22**(29):4578-4580. DOI: 10.1038/sj.onc.1206706

[33] Prete A, Borges de Souza P, Censi S, Muzza M, Nucci N, Sponziello M. Update on fundamental mechanisms of thyroid cancer. Frontiers in Endocrinology (Lausanne). 2020;**11**:102. DOI: 10.3389/fendo.2020.00102

[34] Nikiforov YE, Nikiforova MN. Molecular genetics and diagnosis of thyroid cancer. Nature Reviews. Endocrinology. 2011;**7**(10):569-580. DOI: 10.1038/nrendo.2011.142

[35] Abe I, Lam AK. Anaplastic thyroid carcinoma: Current issues in genomics and therapeutics. Current Oncological Reports. 2021;**23**(3):31. DOI: 10.1007/s11912-021-01019-9

[36] Wu JT, Lin CL, Huang CJ, Cheng YC, Chien CC, Sung YC. Potential synergistic effects of sorafenib and CP-31398 for treating anaplastic thyroid cancer with p53 mutations. Oncology Letters. 2020;**19**(4):3021-3026. DOI: 10.3892/ol.2020.11377

[37] Salvatore D, Santoro M, Schlumberger M. The importance of the RET gene in thyroid cancer and therapeutic implications. Nature Reviews. Endocrinology. 2021;**17**(5):296-306. DOI: 10.1038/s41574-021-00470-9

[38] Xing M. BRAF mutation in papillary thyroid cancer: Pathogenic role, molecular bases, and clinical implications. Endocrine Reviews. 2007;**28**(7):742-762. DOI: 10.1210/er.2007-0007

[39] Khan MS, Qadri Q, Makhdoomi MJ, et al. RET/PTC gene rearrangements in thyroid carcinogenesis: Assessment and Clinico-pathological correlations. Pathology Oncology Research. 2020;**26**(1):507-513. DOI: 10.1007/s12253-018-0540-3

[40] Haroon Al Rasheed MR, Xu B. Molecular alterations in thyroid carcinoma. Surgical Pathological Clinical. 2019;**12**(4):921-930. DOI: 10.1016/j.path.2019.08.002

[41] Borrello MG, Smith DP, Pasini B, et al. RET activation by germline MEN2A and MEN2B mutations. Oncogene. 1995;**11**(11):2419-2427

[42] Accardo G, Conzo G, Esposito D, et al. Genetics of medullary thyroid cancer: An overview. International Journal of Surgery. 2017;**41**(Suppl 1):S2-s6. DOI: 10.1016/j.ijsu.2017.02.064

[43] Enokida T, Tahara M. Management of VEGFR-targeted TKI for thyroid Cancer. Cancers (Basel). 2021;**13**(21):5536. DOI: 10.3390/cancers13215536

[44] Rajabi S, Dehghan MH, Dastmalchi R, Jalali Mashayekhi F, Salami S, Hedayati M. The roles and role-players in thyroid cancer angiogenesis. Endocrinology Journal. 2019;**66**(4):277-293. DOI: 10.1507/endocrj.EJ18-0537

[45] Bunone G, Vigneri P, Mariani L, et al. Expression of angiogenesis stimulators

and inhibitors in human thyroid tumors and correlation with clinical pathological features. The American Journal of Pathology. 1999;**155**(6):1967-1976. DOI: 10.1016/s0002-9440(10)65515-0

[46] Manzella L, Stella S, Pennisi MS, et al. New insights in thyroid cancer and p53 family proteins. International Journal of Molecular Science. 2017;**18**(6):1325. DOI: 10.3390/ijms18061325

[47] Cohen R, Bihan H, Uzzan B, Guetz G, Krivitzky A. Sunitinib and hypothyroidism. Annales d'Endocrinologie (Paris). 2007;**68**(5):332-336. DOI: 10.1016/j.ando.2007.06.027

[48] Ferrari SM, Centanni M, Virili C, et al. Sunitinib in the treatment of thyroid cancer. Current Medicinal Chemistry. 2019;**26**(6):963-972. DOI: 10.2174/0929867324666171006165942

[49] Demlová R, Turjap M, Peš O, Kostolanská K, Juřica J. Therapeutic drug monitoring of Sunitinib in gastrointestinal stromal tumors and metastatic renal cell carcinoma in adults: A review. Therapeutic Drug Monitoring. 2020;**42**(1):20-32. DOI: 10.1097/ftd.0000000000000663

[50] GkountouvasA,Kostoglou-AthanassiouI, Veniou E, Repousis P, Ziras N, Kaldrimidis P. Hematologic toxicity in patients treated with Sunitinib for advanced thyroid cancer. Thyroid. 2010;**20**(6):597-600. DOI: 10.1089/thy.2010.0028

[51] Pasqualetti G, Ricci S, Dardano A, Ferdeghini M, Del Tacca M, Monzani F. The emerging role of sunitinib in the treatment of advanced epithelial thyroid cancer: Our experience and review of literature. Mini Reviews in Medicinal Chemistry. 2011;**11**(9):746-752. DOI: 10.2174/138955711796355249

[52] Kaldrymides P, Kostoglou-Athanassiou I, Gkountouvas A, Veniou E, Ziras N. Partial remission of metastatic papillary thyroid carcinoma with sunitinib. Report of a case and review of the literature. Review Endocrine. 2010;**37**(1):6-10. DOI: 10.1007/s12020-009-9290-z

[53] Ravaud A, de la Fouchardière C, Asselineau J, et al. Efficacy of sunitinib in advanced medullary thyroid carcinoma: Intermediate results of phase II THYSU. Oncologist. 2010;**2010**:212-213

[54] Ravaud A, de la Fouchardière C, Caron P, et al. A multicenter phase II study of sunitinib in patients with locally advanced or metastatic differentiated, anaplastic or medullary thyroid carcinomas: Mature data from the THYSU study. European Journal of Cancer. 2017;**76**:110-117. DOI: 10.1016/j.ejca.2017.01.029

[55] Ferrari SM, Elia G, Ragusa F, et al. Novel treatments for anaplastic thyroid carcinoma. Gland Surgery. 2020;**9**(Suppl 1):S28-s42. DOI: 10.21037/gs.2019.10.18

[56] Fallahi P, Ferrari SM, Santini F, et al. Sorafenib and thyroid cancer. BioDrugs. 2013;**27**(6):615-628. DOI: 10.1007/s40259-013-0049-y

[57] White PT, Cohen MS. The discovery and development of sorafenib for the treatment of thyroid cancer. Expert Opinion Drug Discovery. 2015;**10**(4):427-439. DOI: 10.1517/17460441.2015.1006194

[58] Abdelgalil AA, Alkahtani HM, Al-Jenoobi FI. Sorafenib. Profiles Drug Substances Excip Relation Methodology. 2019;**44**:239-266. DOI: 10.1016/bs.podrm.2018.11.003

[59] Feng G, Luo Y, Zhang Q, Zeng F, Xu J, Zhu J. Sorafenib and radioiodine-refractory differentiated thyroid cancer

(RR-DTC): A systematic review and meta-analysis. Endocrine. 2020;**68**(1): 56-63. DOI: 10.1007/s12020-019-02167-6

[60] Park C, Perini J, Farmer RW, Fancy T, Monga M, Remick SC. Sorafenib and thyroid cancer. Expert Review of Endocrinology and Metabolism. 2014;**9**(6):561-570. DOI: 10.1586/17446651.2014.960391

[61] Chen G, Nicula D, Renko K, Derwahl M. Synergistic anti-proliferative effect of metformin and sorafenib on growth of anaplastic thyroid cancer cells and their stem cells. Oncology Reports. 2015;**33**(4):1994-2000. DOI: 10.3892/or.2015.3805

[62] Zhou M, Zhang G, Hu J, et al. Rutin attenuates Sorafenib-induced Chemoresistance and autophagy in hepatocellular carcinoma by regulating BANCR/miRNA-590-5P/OLR1 Axis. International Journal of Biological Sciences. 2021;**17**(13):3595-3607. DOI: 10.7150/ijbs.62471

[63] Kocaturk NM, Akkoc Y, Kig C, Bayraktar O, Gozuacik D, Kutlu O. Autophagy as a molecular target for cancer treatment. European Journal of Pharmaceutical Sciences. 2019;**134**:116-137. DOI: 10.1016/j.ejps.2019.04.011

[64] Pan H, Wang Z, Jiang L, et al. Autophagy inhibition sensitizes hepatocellular carcinoma to the multikinase inhibitor linifanib. Scientific Reports. 2014;**4**:6683. DOI: 10.1038/srep06683

[65] Cooper MR, Yi SY, Alghamdi W, Shaheen DJ, Steinberg M. Vandetanib for the treatment of medullary thyroid carcinoma. The Annals of Pharmacotherapy. 2014;**48**(3):387-394. DOI: 10.1177/1060028013512791

[66] Fletcher J, Cooper SC, Ghosh S, Hewison M. The role of vitamin D in inflammatory bowel disease: Mechanism to management. Nutrients. 2019;**11**(5):1019. DOI: 10.3390/nu11051019

[67] Ramos HE, Hecht F, Berdelou A, et al. Long-term follow-up and safety of vandetanib for advanced medullary thyroid cancer. Endocrine. 2021;**71**(2):434-442. DOI: 10.1007/s12020-020-02426-x

[68] Leboulleux S, Bastholt L, Krause T, et al. Vandetanib in locally advanced or metastatic differentiated thyroid cancer: A randomised, double-blind, phase 2 trial. The Lancet Oncology. 2012;**13**(9):897-905. DOI: 10.1016/s1470-2045(12)70335-2

[69] Frampton JE. Vandetanib: In medullary thyroid cancer. Drugs. 2012;**72**(10):1423-1436. DOI: 10.2165/11209300-000000000-00000

[70] Tsang VH, Robinson BG, Learoyd DL. The safety of vandetanib for the treatment of thyroid cancer. Expert Opinion on Drug Safety. 2016;**15**(8):1107-1113. DOI: 10.1080/14740338.2016.1201060

[71] Koehler VF, Adam P, Frank-Raue K, et al. Real-world efficacy and safety of Cabozantinib and Vandetanib in advanced medullary thyroid cancer. Thyroid. 2021;**31**(3):459-469. DOI: 10.1089/thy.2020.0206

[72] Suyama K, Iwase H. Lenvatinib: A promising molecular targeted agent for multiple cancers. Cancer Control. 2018;**25**(1):1073. DOI: 10.1177/1073274818789361

[73] Cabanillas ME, Habra MA. Lenvatinib: Role in thyroid cancer and other solid tumors. Cancer Treatment Reviews. 2016;**42**:47-55. DOI: 10.1016/j.ctrv.2015.11.003

[74] Matrone A, Prete A, Nervo A, et al. Lenvatinib as a salvage therapy for advanced metastatic medullary thyroid cancer. Journal of Endocrinological Investigation. 2021;**44**(10):2139-2151. DOI: 10.1007/s40618-020-01491-3

[75] Robinson B, Schlumberger M, Wirth LJ, et al. Characterization of tumor size changes over time from the phase 3 study of Lenvatinib in thyroid Cancer. The Journal of Clinical Endocrinology and Metabolism. 2016;**101**(11):4103-4109. DOI: 10.1210/jc.2015-3989

[76] Takahashi S, Kiyota N, Yamazaki T, et al. A phase II study of the safety and efficacy of lenvatinib in patients with advanced thyroid cancer. Future Oncology. 2019;**15**(7):717-726. DOI: 10.2217/fon-2018-0557

[77] Koyama S, Miyake N, Fujiwara K, et al. Lenvatinib for anaplastic thyroid cancer and Lenvatinib-induced thyroid dysfunction. European Thyroid Journal. 2018;**7**(3):139-144. DOI: 10.1159/000485972

[78] Grüllich C. Cabozantinib: Multi-kinase inhibitor of MET, AXL, RET, and VEGFR2. Recent Results in Cancer Research. 2018;**211**:67-75. DOI: 10.1007/978-3-319-91442-8_5

[79] Elisei R, Schlumberger MJ, Müller SP, et al. Cabozantinib in progressive medullary thyroid cancer. Journal of Clinical Oncology. 2013;**31**(29):3639-3646. DOI: 10.1200/jco.2012.48.4659

[80] Brose MS, Robinson B, Sherman SI, et al. Cabozantinib for radioiodine-refractory differentiated thyroid cancer (COSMIC-311): A randomised, double-blind, placebo-controlled, phase 3 trial. The Lancet Oncology. 2021;**22**(8):1126-1138. DOI: 10.1016/s1470-2045(21)00332-6

[81] Fallahi P, Ferrari SM, Di Bari F, et al. Cabozantinib in thyroid cancer. Recent Patents on Anti-Cancer Drug Discovery. 2015;**10**(3):259-269. DOI: 10.2174/1574892810666150708110816

[82] Schlumberger M, Elisei R, Müller S, et al. Overall survival analysis of EXAM, a phase III trial of cabozantinib in patients with radiographically progressive medullary thyroid carcinoma. Annals of Oncology. 2017;**28**(11):2813-2819. DOI: 10.1093/annonc/mdx479

[83] Knispel S, Zimmer L, Kanaki T, Ugurel S, Schadendorf D, Livingstone E. The safety and efficacy of dabrafenib and trametinib for the treatment of melanoma. Expert Opinion on Drug Safety. 2018;**17**(1):73-87. DOI: 10.1080/14740338.2018.1390562

[84] Subbiah V, Kreitman RJ, Wainberg ZA, et al. Dabrafenib and Trametinib treatment in patients with locally advanced or metastatic BRAF V600-mutant anaplastic thyroid cancer. Journal of Clinical Oncology. 2018;**36**(1):7-13. DOI: 10.1200/jco.2017.73.6785

[85] Subbiah V, Kreitman RJ, Wainberg ZA, et al. Dabrafenib plus trametinib in patients with BRAF V600E-mutant anaplastic thyroid cancer: Updated analysis from the phase II ROAR basket study. Annals of Oncology. 2022;**33**(4):406-415. DOI: 10.1016/j.annonc.2021.12.014

[86] Arıkan R, Telli TA, Demircan NC, et al. Rechallenge with dabrafenib plus trametinib in anaplastic thyroid cancer: A case report and review of literature. Current Problems in Cancer. 2021;**45**(2):100668. DOI: 10.1016/j.currproblcancer.2020.100668

[87] Lorimer C, Cheng L, Chandler R, et al. Dabrafenib and trametinib therapy for advanced anaplastic thyroid

cancer – Real-World Outcomes from UK Centres. Clinical Oncology (R Coll Radiol). 2023;**35**(1):e60-e66. DOI: 10.1016/j.clon.2022.10.017

[88] Markham A. Selpercatinib: First approval. Drugs. 2020;**80**(11):1119-1124. DOI: 10.1007/s40265-020-01343-7

[89] Miyamoto S, Kakutani S, Sato Y, Hanashi A, Kinoshita Y, Ishikawa A. Drug review: Pazopanib. Japanese Journal of Clinical Oncology. 2018;**48**(6):503-513. DOI: 10.1093/jjco/hyy053

[90] Bible KC, Menefee ME, Lin CJ, et al. An international phase 2 study of Pazopanib in progressive and metastatic thyroglobulin antibody negative radioactive iodine refractory differentiated thyroid cancer. Thyroid. 2020;**30**(9):1254-1262. DOI: 10.1089/thy.2019.0269

[91] Cocco E, Scaltriti M, Drilon A. NTRK fusion-positive cancers and TRK inhibitor therapy. Nature Reviews. Clinical Oncology. 2018;**15**(12):731-747. DOI: 10.1038/s41571-018-0113-0

[92] Capdevila J, Awada A, Führer-Sakel D, Leboulleux S, Pauwels P. Molecular diagnosis and targeted treatment of advanced follicular cell-derived thyroid cancer in the precision medicine era. Cancer Treatment Reviews. 2022;**106**:102380. DOI: 10.1016/j.ctrv.2022.102380

[93] Garbe C, Eigentler TK. Vemurafenib. Recent Results in Cancer Research. 2018;**211**:77-89. DOI: 10.1007/978-3-319-91442-8_6

[94] Semsar-Kazerooni K, Morand GB, Payne AE, et al. Mutational status may supersede tumor size in predicting the presence of aggressive pathologic features in well differentiated thyroid cancer. Journal of Otolaryngology Head and Neck Surgery. 2022;**51**(1):9. DOI: 10.1186/s40463-022-00559-9

Chapter 6

Aspects Considered in Differentiated Thyroid Cancer for Radioiodine Therapy

Aisyah Elliyanti

Abstract

Thyroid cancer incidence has rapidly increased in high-income countries for the past 30 years. The increase in thyroid cancer cases may be due to improved diagnostic methods or exposure to unknown risk factors. Even though new thyroid cancer cases have increased, the mortality rate is relatively stable. Most thyroid cancer is differentiated thyroid cancer (DTC). Conventional management of DTC consists of near-total thyroidectomy followed by ablation therapy with radioiodine-131 (RAI). RAI was first used nearly 80 years ago to treat thyroid cancer and still plays a pivotal role in managing DTC. There are three RAI therapy options: remnant ablation, adjuvant therapy, and known disease treatments. After thyroid resection, radioactive Iodine-131 (RAI) is recommended for patients with intermediate to high risk of recurrent disease or distant metastases. Long-term follow-up is needed to detect a persistence or recurrence of the disease after initial RAI administration. RAI effectively improves treatment efficiency and reduces the risk of cancer recurrence and metastasis post-thyroid resection. Clinical outcome prediction is ultimately defined by appropriate management. This article will review some factors to consider when planning RAI therapy for DTC and subsequent surveillance after the therapy.

Keywords: adjuvant therapy, remnant ablation, refractory thyroid, risk- stratification, serum thyroglobulin, whole body scan

1. Introduction

Thyroid cancer is a malignant endocrine tumor [1]. Papillary thyroid cancer (PTC) and follicular thyroid cancer (FTC) are classified as differentiated thyroid cancer (DTC), which is approximately 95% of all thyroid carcinomas [2, 3]. Over the past 30 years, the incidence of DTC has rapidly increased worldwide [3–6]. The increase in thyroid cancer cases may be due to improved diagnostic methods or exposure to unknown risk factors [1, 5, 6]. Conversely to the increase of new cases, the mortality rates have been steadily declining in most areas of the world [7, 8]. The condition is likely due to improved diagnostic methods, management, and treatment of the disease [7, 8]. DTC is considered a slow-growing malignancy with a generally good prognosis with 5-year survival for the localized disease at 99.9% and for regional metastatic disease at 97.8% [4, 6]. However, distant metastatic DTC is associated with a significantly worse prognosis (5-year survival of 55.3% [4, 6].

After resection of DTC, conventional management is followed by the administration of radioactive Iodine-131 (RAI) in most patients for both thyroid remnant ablation and treatment of expected or proven locoregional or distant metastases [1, 2]. Thyroid follicular cells take up and accumulate radioiodine, the same process as iodine, except for organification [9]. The process utilizes the expression of sodium iodide symporter (NIS), thyroglobulin (Tg), thyroid stimulating hormone receptor (TSHR), thyroperoxidase (TPO), and thyroid-specific transcription factors (bone gene-8 (PAX-8), thyroid transcription factor-1 (TTF-1)) [10]. Even though thyroid cancer cells, including metastases, take up RAI, the efficacy of RAI is limited in large tumor sizes, which need to be treated repeatedly [1, 2, 11, 12]. A study reported a decreased risk of death and risk of recurrence for tumors > 1 cm in a group of 269 patients with PTC treated with extensive initial surgery and then RAI remnant ablation [2]. Moreover, RAI treatment is recommended in high-risk and intermediate-risk patients, where the decision should be on an individual and tumor features basis [1, 2, 11]. This chapter's objective is to discuss the indication of radioiodine therapy in DTC.

2. Iodine and radioiodine transport

Radioiodine is the first radionuclide used for therapy in clinical oncology, including thyroid cancer therapy. It is a beta (β) and gamma (γ) emitter that is used for therapy and also for imaging [9, 13, 14]. RAI is administrated in the form of liquid or a capsule. Once it is ingested, it is quickly absorbed into the bloodstream from the gastrointestinal (GI) tract. Thyroid follicular cells take up RAI through active transport, regulated by thyroid-stimulating hormone (TSH), which requires energy produced by ouabain-sensitive Na^+/K^+-adenosine triphosphatase (Na^+/K^+-ATPase) using the NIS as co-transport [9, 15, 16]. About 20% of the ingested iodine is converted to iodide (I^-) before being absorbed [17]. In plasma, there is an exchange of iodide with red blood cells and extracellular compartments. The thyroid gland collects as much as 70–90% of I^- in the body [18]. Besides being captured by the thyroid gland, iodide is collected in the salivary glands, gastric mucosa, choroid plexus, and breast glands and enters the placental circulation. The thyroid gland can collect I^- as much as 20–40 times compared with plasma under normal physiological conditions [19, 20].

3. Pathology and molecular markers of differentiated thyroid cancer

The main histopathology types of thyroid cancer (TC) consist of papillary and follicular, poorly differentiated (PDTC), anaplastic thyroid cancer (ATC), and medullary thyroid cancer (MTC) from the C cells [21–23]. Papillary thyroid cancer (PTC) and follicular thyroid cancer (FTC) are two distinct histological forms of the DTC type [2]. PTC patients are typically younger than 50 and have smaller tumors, a higher incidence of lymph node metastases, multi-centricity, and extra-thyroidal extension. Patients with FTC show a higher incidence of distant metastatic disease and more frequently receive repeated radioiodine [2]. Tumor pathologies show significant variability among the tumors. The variation is particularly notable among types originating from thyroid follicular cells. The progression of DTC to PDTC and ATC is most likely the result of additional genetic mutations developing after the primary oncogenic event, which provides the tumor with a more aggressive growth initiative. Alternatively, the cancer phenotype may be dictated by the differential nature of the stem cells capable of initiating PTC, FTC, and ATC [24]. The most common thyroid cancer mutations originate from follicular or parafollicular cells [25]. These mutations are the basis for the design of molecular markers and molecular approaches to thyroid cancer.

In some populations, malignant DTC might only occasionally lead to death, including cases of PTC in children and young adults presenting with lymph node metastases (LNMs). Some TC types were recently reclassified from malignant to benign, such as noninvasive follicular thyroid neoplasm with papillary-like nuclear features (NIFTP) [21]. Based on clinical evidence, it is associated with no reports of cancer-related deaths and estimated risk of recurrence of <1% [26]. PTC accounts for 80% of TC with molecular characteristics predominant consisting of BRAF mutation, RAS mutation, and RET rearrangements, nearly 70% as shown in **Table 1** [28]. These mutations are

Classification	Tumor types	Markers
Benign	Follicular adenoma	RAS, PAX8/PPARγ, PI3K/AKT
Borderline/uncertain	Hyalinizing trabecular tumor other encapsulated follicular patterned tumors • Follicular tumor of UMP • Well-diffrentiated tumor of UMP • NIFT-P	RAS, BRAF
Malignant	PTC • Papillary carcinoma • Follicular variant of PTC • Encapsulated variant of PTC • Papillary micro-carcinoma • Columnar cell variant of PTC • Oncocytic variant of PT	BRAF (40–50%) RAS (15%) RET/PTC (20–40%) PAX8/PPARγ (rare)
	FTC • Minimally invasive • Encapsulated angioinvasive • Widely invasive	RAS (20–40%) PAX8/PPARγ (10–66%) PI3K/AKT (rare)
	Hurthle cell carcinoma Capsular invasion, Vascular invasion >4 blood	RAS, EIF1AX, TP53, CNA, mtDNA
	Poorly differentiated thyroid carcinoma	TERT (42%) BRAF (32%) RAS (19%)
	Anaplastic thyroid carcinoma	TP53 (60%) TERT (33%) BRAF (56%)

Uncertain Malignant Potential (UMP)
Non-Invasive Follicular Thyroid neoplasm with Papillary-like nuclear features (NIFT-P). References: [10, 22, 32].

Table 1.
Classification of thyroid cancer based on World Health Organization (WHO) 2017.

associated with radioiodine refractory (RAIR) [10]. BRAF ^{V600E} mutations are frequently reported in a subgroup of PTCs with more aggressive behavior [23, 26, 28–30]. The fatal forms of non-anaplastic cancer are generally PTC variants harboring BRAF or RAS mutations plus other genomic alterations such as mutations involving the TERT promoter, POLE, TP53, PI3K/AKT/mTOR pathway, SWI/SNF subunits, and/or histone methyltransferases [10, 30, 31]. BRAF mutations are present in 30%–67% of PTCs and are associated with locoregional metastases and extra-thyroidal extension [32]. A positive test for BRAF mutations means a close to 100% probability of malignancy [27]. This is likely helpful to guide the extent of thyroidectomy.

Follicular thyroid, accounting for 2%–5% of TC cancer, is considered minimally invasive when capsular penetration is present without vascular involvement (a condition associated with an excellent prognosis) by WHO [10, 11]. The angioinvasive and widely invasive term is when neoplastic emboli involve < 4 or ≥ 4 blood vessels, respectively [11]. FTC type is frequently linked to activation of the PI3K and MAPK pathways through loss of PTEN expression, NRAS mutations, rearrangements such as PPARγ/PAX8, and other events [27, 28, 30]. Hurthle cell carcinomas are no longer classified as follicular tumors. They are generally much less aggressive and less likely to present with lymph node metastases [11]. Hurthle cell carcinomas associated with extensive vascular and/or capsular invasion should be managed like other high-risk carcinomas [11].

Furthermore, once thyroid cancer is highly suspected or diagnosed, a decision must be made regarding the extent of surgery. Risk factors must be considered, such as clinical risk factors associated with aggressive tumor behavior, the patient's age and sex, the initial tumor size and location, the presence of lymph nodes and/or distant metastases, cytologic and mutational data, and patient preferences. Most DTC can be identified through cytology, and when the result is indeterminate, assessment with malignancy markers (HBME1 or galectin-3) and molecular alterations (BRAF mutations, RET fusions, other novel gene alterations) are reportedly helpful for identifying malignancy [11].

4. Risk stratification

Accurate staging and assessment of DTC risk are essential for its management, which determines the prognosis and guides therapeutic decisions and the intensity of surveillance [4]. Risk stratification in DTC was based on clinic-pathological features after a few weeks of completing thyroidectomy, which previously referred to a static estimate of disease-specific mortality. Nowadays, risk stratification is a dynamic, active process used to predict the appropriateness of minimalistic initial therapy, risk of recurrence, disease-specific mortality, and the most likely response to initial treatment, as shown in **Table 2**. Moreover, an excellent histopathology report is essential for proper risk stratification [1, 11]. The estimated risk of recurrence ranges from <1% to 55%, and it is classified as low if ≤ 5%, intermediate if 6%–20%, and high if >20%, based on the presence or absence of aggressive features, presence of local or distant metastases, and imaging features on whole-body post-therapy scans [1, 2, 11]

Several systems are designed for risk stratification, considering patients' age, tumor size, resection completeness, local invasion, and distant metastasis [12]. The DTC risk stratification is applied in the clinical setting despite a validated system's absence [12, 33]. The original ATA risk category design (low, intermediate, high) is usually applied in clinical practice with promising results [12]. However, the 2015

ATA risk stratification system was built on retrospective studies where nearly all patients were treated with RAI. ATA risk stratification schema for selecting patients for adjuvant treatment is not conclusively validated. However, it prompts the physician to consider the various clinic-pathologic factors in managing low- intermediate-risk patients where the indication for RAI therapy may not be straightforward [1]. The initial risk stratification is revised during follow-up to evaluate the disease and treatment responses (dynamic risk stratification) because the biological behavior of the disease as a response to therapy was not accounted for in initial staging [11, 12].

5. Radioiodine therapy (RAIT)

The ability of thyroid follicular cell to take up and concentrate iodide becomes the basic fundamental of RAI therapy. Selecting the appropriate method for RAI treatment requires careful evaluation of postoperative status. However, no universally accepted recommendations exist to assess postoperative disease status [34]. Consensus in 2019 of the American Thyroid Association (ATA), the European Association of Nuclear Medicine and Molecular Imaging (EANM), the Society of Nuclear Medicine and Molecular Imaging (SNMMI), and the European Thyroid Association (ETA) state that the goal of the administration of RAIT in differentiated thyroid cancer is for remnant ablation, adjuvant treatment for irradiation of resumed foci of tumor cells to reduce the recurrence risk, or treat persistent or recurrent disease [1, 11, 12]. Remnant ablation is done after near/total thyroidectomy to destroy presumably benign residual thyroid tissue to eliminate thyroglobulin (Tg) production, facilitating follow-up of remnant ablation [1, 11, 12]. The adjuvant treatment goal is to eliminate potential microscopic foci of thyroid cancer tissue after complete resection of thyroid metastatic (locoregional, distant, or both). The condition can minimize the risk of recurrence, improving disease-specific and progression-free survival. Treatment of persistent or recurrent disease aims to improve progression-free, disease-specific, and overall survival at radioiodine-avid DTC, where the diagnosis is based on anatomical detection or biochemical evidence [1, 11, 12].

A joint of the ATA, the SNMMI, the EANM, and the ETA published a statement acknowledging the absence of high-quality evidence against using RAIT for remnant ablation post-total thyroidectomy for low-risk patients, and RAIT decisions should be taken on an individual basis, depending on tumor features (risk of recurrence), patient-related factors (comorbidities, motivation, emotional concerns), healthcare setting (availability and quality of thyroid surgeons, ultrasonography, RAI scintigraphy, Tg assays), and the local management preferences [11]. The benefit of RAIT should outweigh the risks associated with its administration, which include adverse events and diminished quality of life (QoL) [1, 11]. Application of RAIT activity dose has three broad approaches [4]: (1). Empiric dose (based on convention, experience, and patient-related factors. (2). A maximum permissible dose (determined by the upper bound limit of whole-body blood [bone marrow] dosimetry (WBBD)). (3). Target/lesion dosimetry. ATA guidelines do not endorse RAI dose activity one over the other [2, 12]. The level of risk for persistent/recurrent disease will determine the RAI dose activities. A ^{131}I-whole-body scan (^{131}I-WBS) must follow RAI administration to document the RAI avidity and stage of the disease [12]. ^{131}I-WBS post-therapy scans may show additional metastases in 10–26% of patients compared with pre-therapy scans [35, 36]. Extensive disease noted on ^{131}I-WBS post-therapy may alter the clinical stage in about 10% and clinical management in 10–15% of DTC patients [2].

Level of risk	Histology	Definition	RAI therapy (ATA recommendation)	RAI doses (ATA recommendation)
Low ≤5%	NFTP	Noninvasive follicular thyroid tumor with papillary-like nuclear features ('non-invasive encapsulated follicular-variant PTC)'		
	PTC	With all of the following: • Without macroscopic tumor remnants • Without loco-regional invasion or local metastases • Clinical N0 or pathology N1 (<5 micrometastases, each <0.2 cm) • Without distant metastases • No RAI uptake shown outside the thyroid bed on post-treatment whole-body RAI scan (if available) • Without vascular invasion • Non-aggressive histology BRAF V600E-mutated PTCs can is assigned to the low-risk if the tumor is <1 cm	Remnant ablation is not routinely recommended, unless aggressive histology or vascular invasion. Other factors may also be considered	1.11 GBq (30 mCi) if given to patients without aggressive histology or vascular invasion
	FTC	Intrathyroidal, well-differentiated FTC with capsular invasion and minimal (<4 foci) or without vascular invasion		
Intermediate (6%–20%)	PTC	With at least one of the following: • Microscopic invasion of perithyroidal soft tissues • Tumor-related symptoms • Intra-thyroidal tumor measuring <4cm, BRAFV600E-mutated (if available) • Aggressive histology • Vascular invasion • Multifocal papillary micro carcinoma with extra thyroid extension (ETE) and known BRAFV600E mutation • Clinical N1or pathological N1 (>5 involved lymph nodes, each measuring <3 cm) • RAI uptake of metastatic foci in the neck on the first post-therapy RAI WBS.	Consider adjuvant therapy with consideration of risk of recurrent disease, especially in tumors >2 cm, histology, vascular invasion and, potentially other factors. Advancing age (≥ 45 or 55) favors for RAI therapy	>1.11 GBq up to 55.5 GBq (>30 up to 150 mCi)
	FTC	With at least one of the following: • Clinical N1 or pathological N1 disease (>5 involved lymph nodes, each measuring <3 cm) • RAI- WBS shown metastatic foci uptake in the neck post RAI therapy		

DOI: http://dx.doi.org/10.5772/intechopen.108481

Level of risk	Histology	Definition	RAI therapy (ATA recommendation)	RAI doses (ATA recommendation)
High (>20%)	PTC	With at least one of the following: • Gross ETE (macroscopic invasion of peri-thyroidal soft tissues) • Pathological N1: one or more nodal metastases measuring> 3 cm. • Extra nodal extension • Concomitant BRAFV600E and TERT mutations • Postoperative serum Tg suggestive of distant metastases • Incomplete tumor resection • Distant metastases	Adjuvant treatment is recommended	>1.11 GBq up to 55.5GBq
	FTC	With at least one of the following: • Widely invasive or extensive vascular invasion(>4foci) • Postoperative serum Tg suggestive of distant metastases • Incomplete tumor resection • Distant metastases		

References: [1, 10].

Table 2.
Risk stratification and recommendation of radioiodine therapy.

The RAI activity consists of low and high doses. A low dose is usually given for remnant ablation at 1.1 GBq (30 mCi) [1, 11]. A high dose for treatment at > 1.1 GBq–5.55 GBq (>30 mCi–150 mCi), is recommended for high-risk recurrence conditions as shown in **Table 2** [1, 11, 12, 37]. The RAIT is not recommended for particular low-risk/very low-risk conditions [tumor with a small size nodule (< 1cm intrathyroidal) and without locoregional metastases] [11]. The administered RAI activities higher than 5.55 GBq (150 mCi) are unnecessary in intermediate-risk patients. Limiting RAI dose activities to a maximal 5.55 GBq (150 mCi) mainly considers the risks of side effects [1]. Regarding the treatment of known DTC, the ATA guidelines recommend RAI dose up to 7.40 GBq (200 mCi) and not to exceed 5.55 GBq (150 mCi) in patients ≥70 years old, to avoid the risk of toxicity [12]. In patients with prolonged radioiodine clearance, the RAI dose is reduced by up to 50% [38, 39].

Parameters	Excellent	Biochemical incomplete	Structural incomplete	Indeterminate
1. Serum Tg				
• Non-stimulated	< 0.2 ng/ml	≥ 1 ng/ml	Any	0.2 to < 1ng/ml
• Stimulated	<1 ng/ml	≥10ng/ml	Any	1 to < 10ng/ml
2. Anti-Tg antibody	Undetectable	Increasing	Any	Stable or decreasing
3. Imaging results	Negative	Negative	Residual disease positive	Equivocal
4. Prognosis	1%–4% recurrence	Without evidence (spontaneously ≈30%, after additional treatment ≈20%).	Persistent disease (50%–85%)	Stable or resolves in ≈ 80% Response is reclassified as structural or biochemical incomplete and may need additional therapy in ≈20%
5. Disease-specific mortality	< 1%	< 1%	Loco-regional metastasis up to 11%; and distant metastasis up to 57%	< 1%
6. Response based on classification				
• Low	86% to 91%	11% to 19%	2% to 6 %	12% to 29%
• Intermediate	57% to 63%	21% to 22%	19% to 28%	8 % to 23%
• High	14% to 16%	16% to 18%	67% to 75%	0.5 to 4%

References: [10, 11].

Table 3.
Treatment responses of differentiated thyroid cancer treated with total thyroidectomy and radioiodine therapy.

In low-risk DTC patients, RAIT is influenced by any adverse feature that modulates recurrence risk and patient preference. The ATA 2015 guidelines recommend a low RAI dose (1.11 GBq/30 mCi) for remnant ablation of low-risk or intermediate-risk DTC with low-risk features [2, 11, 12]. Radioiodine therapy after total thyroidectomy should be considered in intermediate-risk DTC and is routinely recommended in ATA high-risk DTC. The therapy consideration is to balance treatment efficacy with unwanted side effects [1]. However, patient preference plays a crucial role in decision-making. Therefore, the activity of RAI ought to be specifically prescribed for each patient [12]. Moreover, on the 2015 ATA guidelines, RAI for adjuvant therapy is considered for DTC having a low-to-intermediate risk for recurrence with (1). Tumor with a dimension > 4 cm without nodal or distant metastases (T3a N0 or Nx M0 or Mx) by the AJCC 8th edition, TNM classification. (2). Any tumor size with microscopic extra-thyroidal extension but without nodal or distant metastasis (3). Tumors (T1–T3a) with nodal but no distant metastasis (T1–T3a N1 M0 or Mx) (4). Tumors (T1–T3a) with vascular invasion and aggressive pathological subtype [1, 11]. A microscopic residual disease increases in intermediate-risk DTC, as evidenced by higher recurrence rates in most intermediate categories compared with low-risk. A study that reported adjuvant RAIT in intermediate-risk patients with the exclusion of aggressive variants and multiple primaries showed a survival benefit in patients <45 years old, and improved overall survival was also shown in patients with aggressive variants of PTC [40–42]. The adjuvant therapy of RAI in high-risk DTC without distant metastasis shows improved outcome and without controversial decision. RAI adjuvant therapy is recommended in patients with T3b, T4a, and T4b, any N, M0, and high-risk DTC, including cervical nodes (≥3 cm in largest dimension) and/or with extranodal extension [1]. Treatment responses after total thyroidectomy and RAIT are defined as excellent, biochemical incomplete, structural incomplete, or indeterminate based on findings (neck ultrasound and serum Tg and anti-Tg anti- body (TgAb) levels, as shown in **Table 3**.

6. Radioiodine refractory (RAI refractory)

DTC cells can retain functions of follicular cells, such as iodide uptake and iodination, which allows RAI uptake for treating cancer [43]. Most DTC cases have a favorable prognosis after standard therapy, including total thyroidectomy, selective RAI therapy, and TSH suppressive therapy. NIS plays a role in the active transport of iodide into the thyroid follicular cells [9]. Functional NIS expression is regulated at the transcriptional and posttranslational levels, and TSH is primarily involved at the translational level [43]. Concerning posttranslational regulation, abundant NIS expression may mislocalize in the intracellular compartment rather than the cell membrane [43]. This mislocation targeting of NIS disturbs uptake and accumulation of radioiodine, inducing the failure of RAI therapy in DTC [10, 43]. The local recurrence and distant metastasis risk increase to 20% and 10%, respectively [10]. Among these cases, two-thirds show initial or gradual loss of the ability of iodine uptake due to the dysfunction, and even loss, of NIS expression in the basal membrane, indicating a status of dedifferentiation known as radioiodine-refractory (RAIR), which significantly reduces the 10-year survival rate less than 10% [9, 43].

Radioiodine refractory is when progressive dedifferentiation of the tumor cells leads to a loss of ability to accumulate RAI by non-functioning the sodium iodide symporter [43, 44]. The condition included is (a) tumor or metastatic site (one or multiple) that does not ever concentrate radioiodine (no avidity outside the thyroid bed on the initial post-therapy WBS); (b) tumor tissue that initially showed RAI avidity but lost the ability to concentrate on subsequent scans or treatments; (c) radioiodine is concentrated in some, but not all, sites of metastatic; (d) disease progression despite significant concentration of RAI (within 1 year of treatment) [10, 44].

Decreased NIS expression, diminished membrane targeting, or both, which are mainly caused by genetic and epigenetic alterations and dysregulated signaling pathways, are the primary mechanisms underlying RAIR [10]. Genetic alterations in MAPK and phosphoinositide 3-kinase (PI3K)/AKT signaling pathways by point mutations or chromosomal rearrangements are basic molecules in the pathogenesis of thyroid cancers and RAIR. Besides the signaling pathways, epigenetic and genetic alterations of other pathways, such as Wnt/ß-catenin and TGF-ß/Smad signaling pathways, are also related to the silencing of expression of thyroid-specific genes, resulting in RAIR [10, 28].

The evidence has demonstrated a strong association between the *BRAF*^{V600E} mutation and RAI-avidity loss in PTC [43]. The *BRAF*^{V600E} mutation can upregulate the expression of tumor-promoting genes, such as *TGFβ1,* mesenchymal-to-epithelial transition factor [*MET*], vascular endothelial growth factor A [*VEGFA*], and thrombospondin 1 [*TSP1*]) [43, 45]. It can downregulate the expression genes of tumor suppressors such as tissue inhibitor of metalloproteinases 3 [*TIMP3*], death-associated protein kinase 1 [*DAPK1*]), and solute carrier family five-member 8 [*SLC5A8]*, [46]. *BRAF*^{V600E} mutation induces the secretion of TGFβ, which can stimulate SMAD3 and impair PAX8, which cause a decrease in NIS expression [43]. Moreover, telomerase reverse transcriptase (*TERT*) promoter (TERTp) mutations are particularly prevalent in *BRAF*^{V600E} mutation PTC. TERTp mutations were associated with aggressive tumor behavior and poor prognosis in thyroid cancer. They were also observed to be correlated with the reduction of RAI uptake in distant metastatic lesions of PTC [10, 43]. On the other hand, the RET/PTC rearrangement impacts the dedifferentiation of DTC remains limited. In vitro studies reported that alternation of RET/PTC could suppress the expression of thyroid differentiation markers (TPO, TSH receptor, thyroglobulin, and NIS) [47, 48]. Recently, oncogene-activated signaling pathways have also been reported to control histone posttranslational modification affecting thyroid-specific genes' expression [10, 49]. This finding supports attempts to convert thyroid cancer into redifferentiated thyroid cancer by modulating histone acetylation and deacetylation [10, 43]. *BRAF*-activated NIS silencing could be influenced by histone deacetylation at critical regulatory regions of the *NIS* promoter [10].

7. Patient preparation

The effectiveness of RAIT depends on patient preparation. Ideally, serum TSH levels reach ≥30 mU/L to optimize radioiodine uptake [50]. TSH elevation can be reached by waiting at least 3 weeks after thyroidectomy or 4–5 weeks after discontinuing treatment with levothyroxine (LT4). When thyroid hormone is withheld, it should be initiated or resumed 2 days after radioiodine administration [50]. Recombinant human thyrotropin (rhTSH) administration is an acceptable alternative to thyroid hormone withdrawal (TWH) based on ATA guidelines before remnant ablation or adjuvant treatment in low-risk and intermediate-risk DTC without extensive lymph node involvement. In extensive lymph node disease without distant metastasis, the rhTSH stimulation may be considered an alternative to THW before

RAIT. The rhTSH is not approved yet by Food and Drug Administration (FDA) to treat distant metastases of DTC. The rhTSH stimulation is recommended for any patient with DTC regardless of the risk level if comorbidities exist that preclude THW [12]. Furthermore, patients should be advised to avoid iodine-containing medications (iodinated contrast agents, antiseptics, eye drops or amiodarone, and iodine-containing foods) for 4–6 weeks prior to RAIT to avoid competition with non-radioactive iodine. Moreover, a low-iodine diet (<50 μg/day), starting 1– 2 weeks prior to RAIT, is recommended optionally [50]. Patients are advised to avoid meals for at least 2 hours before and 2 hours after administering RAI because heavy meals can slow the absorption of RAI [16].

8. Follow-ups

The follow-ups are carried out every 6 months (for the first 5 years after diagnosis), and if no pathological findings since the period, examinations are adequate annually [49, 51]. The follow-up assessment is based on the interview, clinical examination, cervical sonography, and determination of TSH and thyroid hormone levels, Tg, and Tg antibodies. When postoperative hypoparathyroidism occurs, substitution therapy is needed. A diagnostic WBS is obligatory 6–12 months after the initial RAIT, and the next WBS is needed if there is a relapse indication [12, 52]. Metastatic uptake on ^{131}I-WBS confirms their capacity to concentrate RAI and the potential to respond to RAI in this condition as a permit for RAI activity to treat metastases.

The criteria for a disease-free (6–12 months) after initial therapy of DTC with total thyroidectomy and RAIT are no clinical signs of DTC and without pathological uptake in ^{131}I-WBS (except the uptake showed after remnant ablation). A serum Tg is below the detection limit, and undetected Tg antibodies [12, 52]. In conditions with elevated/rising Tg serum levels and undetectable radioiodine uptake, F-18-fluorodeoxyglucose positron emission tomography (^{18}FDG-PET) examination is recommended [49, 50, 53].

9. Conclusions

The RAI administration aims at remnant ablation and adjuvant treatment for irradiating presumed foci of tumor cells to reduce the recurrence risk or treat persistent or recurrent disease. The risk stratification after thyroidectomy becomes pivotal in DTC management to offer an individualized therapy approach. The decisions should be taken depending on tumor features, patient-related factors, healthcare settings, and local team preferences. The local team was considered by interdisciplinary teams in the initial management of DTC patients, focusing on RAIT. Even though RAIT in the low-intermediate risk class is still debatable, RAIT is recommended in high-risk DTC without distant metastasis, showing improved outcomes and without controversial decisions.

Conflict of interest

The author has no possible conflict of interest.

Author details

Aisyah Elliyanti
Nuclear Medicine Division of Radiology, Department Faculty of Medicine,
Universitas Andalas/Dr. M.Djamil Hospital, Padang, Indonesia

*Address all correspondence to: aelliyanti@med.unand.ac.id

References

[1] Juweid ME, Tulchinsky M, Mismar A, Momani M, Zayed AA, Al Hawari H, et al. Contemporary considerations in adjuvant radioiodine treatment of adults with differentiated thyroid cancer. International Journal of Cancer. 2020;**147**:2345-2354

[2] Grewal RK, Ho A, Schöder H. Novel approaches to thyroid cancer treatment and response assessment. Seminars in Nuclear Medicine. 2016;**46**:109-118

[3] Lorusso L, Cappagli V, Valerio L, Giani C, Viola D, Puleo L, et al. Thyroid cancers: From surgery to current and future systemic therapies through their molecular identities. International Journal of Molecular Sciences. 2021;**22**:3117

[4] Donohoe KJ, Aloff J, Avram AM, Bennet KG, Giovanella L, Greenspan B, et al. Appropriate use criteria for nuclear medicine in the evaluation and treatment of differentiated thyroid cancer. Journal of Nuclear Medicine. 2020;**61**:375-396

[5] American Thyroid Association (ATA) Guidelines Taskforce on Thyroid Nodules and Differentiated Thyroid Cancer, Cooper DS, Doherty GM, Haugen BR, Kloos RT, Lee SL, et al. Revised American Thyroid Association management guidelines for patients with thyroid nodules and differentiated thyroid cancer. Thyroid. 2009;**19**:1167-1214

[6] Olson E, Wintheiser G, Wolfe KM, Droessler J, Silberstein PT. Epidemiology of thyroid cancer: A review of the national cancer database, 2000-2013. Cureus. 2019;**11**:e4127

[7] Seib CD, Sosa JA. Evolving understanding of the epidemiology of thyroid cancer. Endocrinology and Metabolism Clinics of North America. 2019;**48**:23-35

[8] La Vecchia C, Malvezzi M, Bosetti C, Garavello W, Bertuccio P, et al. Thyroid cancer mortality and incidence: A global overview. International Journal of Cancer. 2015;**136**:2187-2195

[9] Salih S, Alkatheeri A, Alomaim W, Elliyanti A. Radiopharmaceutical treatments for cancer therapy, radionuclides characteristics, applications, and challenges. Molecules. 2022;**16**:5231

[10] Oh JM, Ahn BC. Molecular mechanisms of radioactive iodine refractoriness in differentiated thyroid cancer: Impaired sodium iodide symporter (NIS) expression owing to altered signaling pathway activity and intracellular localization of NIS. Theranostics. 2021;**11**(13):6251-6277

[11] Filetti S, Durante C, Hartl D, Leboulleux S, Locati LD, Newbold K, et al. Thyroid cancer: ESMO Clinical Practice Guidelines for diagnosis, treatment and follow-up†. Annals of Oncology. 2019;**30**:1856-1883

[12] Ciarallo A, Rivera J. Radioactive iodine therapy in differentiated thyroid cancer: 2020 update. AJR. American Journal of Roentgenology. 2020;**215**:285-291

[13] Elliyanti A. Radiopharmaceuticals in modern cancer therapy. In: Badria FA, editor. Radiopharmaceutical Current Research for Better Diagnosis, Therapy, Environmental and Pharmaceutical Applications. 1st ed. London, UK, London, United Kingdom: Intechopen; 2021

[14] Elliyanti A. Molecular radiobiology and radionuclides therapy concepts.

In: Jekunen A, editor. The Evolutionof Radionanotargeting towards Clinical Precission Oncology: A Festschrift in Honor of Kalevi Kairemo. UAE: Bentham Science; 2022. pp. 395-408

[15] Elliyanti A, Rusnita D, Afriani N, Susanto YD, et al. Analysis natrium iodide symporter expression in breast cancer sub-types for radioiodine therapy response. Nuclear Medicine and Molecular Imaging. 2020;**54**:35-42

[16] Elliyanti A. Radioiodine for Graves' disease therapy. In: Gensure R, editor. Graves' Diseas. 1st ed. London: Intechopen; 2021

[17] Cavalieri RR. Iodine metabolism and thyroid physiology: Current concepts. Thyroid. 1997;**7**(2):177-181

[18] Kogai TBG. The sodium iodide symporter (NIS): Regulation and approaches to targeting for cancer therapeutics. Pharmacology & Therapeutics. 2012;**135**:355-370

[19] De La Vieja A, Dohan O, Levy O, Carrasco N. Molecular analysis of the sodium/iodide symporter: Impact on thyroid and extrathyroid pathophysiology. Physiological Reviews. 2000;**80**(3):1083-1105

[20] Dohan O, De la Vieja A, Paroder V, Riedel C, Artani M, Reed M, et al. The sodium/iodide Symporter (NIS): Characterization, regulation, and medical significance. Endocrine Reviews. 2003;**24**:48-77

[21] Chmielik E, Rusinek D, Oczko-Wojciechowska M, Jarzab M, Krajewska J, et al. Heterogeneity of thyroid cancer. Pathobiology. 2018;**85**:117-129

[22] Asa SL. The current histologic classification of thyroid cancer. Endocrinology and Metabolism Clinics of North America. 2019;**48**:1-22

[23] Wells SA, Santoro M. Update: The status of clinical trials with kinase inhibitors in thyroid cancer. The Journal of Clinical Endocrinology and Metabolism. 2014;**99**:1543-1555

[24] Todaro M, Iovino F, Eterno V, et al. Tumorigenic and metastatic activity of human thyroid cancer stem cells. Cancer Research. 2010;**70**:8874-8885

[25] Nikiforov YE, Nikiforova MN. Molecular genetics and diagnosis of thyroid cancer. Nature Reviews. Endocrinology. 2011;**7**:569-580

[26] Pacini F, Basolo F, Bellantone R, et al. Italian consensus on diagnosis and treatment of differentiated thyroid cancer: Joint statements of six Italian societies. Journal of Endocrinological Investigation. 2018;**41**:849-876

[27] Nikiforov YE, Yip L, Nikiforova MN. New strategies in diagnosing cancer in thyroid nodules: Impact of molecular markers. Clinical Cancer Research. 2013;**19**:2283-2288

[28] Prete A et al. Update on fundamental mechanisms of thyroid cancer. Frontiers in Endocrinology. 2020;**11**:102

[29] Brierley JD, Gospodarowicz MK, Wittekind C. UICC TNM Classification of Malignant Tumours. 8th ed. Oxford: John Wiley & Sons Inc; 2016

[30] Xing M. Molecular pathogenesis and mechanisms of thyroid cancer. Nature Reviews. Cancer. 2013;**13**:184-199

[31] Ibrahimpasic T, Xu B, Landa I, et al. Genomic alterations in fatal forms of non-anaplastic thyroid cancer: Identification of MED12 and RBM10 as novel thyroid cancer genes associated

with tumor virulence. Clinical Cancer Research. 2017;**23**:5970-5980

[32] Raue F, Frank-Raue K. Thyroid cancer: Risk-stratified management and individualized therapy. Clinical Cancer Research. 2016;**22**:5012-5021

[33] Tuttle RM, Alzahrani AS. Risk stratification in differentiated thyroid cancer: From detection to final follow-up. The Journal of Clinical Endocrinology and Metabolism. 2019;**104**:4087-4100

[34] Tuttle RM, Ahuja S, Avram AM, et al. Controversies, consensus, and collaboration in the use of 131I therapy in differentiated thyroid cancer: A joint statement from the American Thyroid Associa tion, the European Association of Nuclear Medicine, the Society of Nuclear Medicine and Molecular Imaging, and the European Thyroid Association. Thyroid. 2019;**29**:461-470

[35] Fatourechi V, Hay ID, Mullan BP, et al. Are posttherapy radioiodine scans informative and do they influence subsequent therapy of patients with differentiated thyroid cancer? Thyroid: Official Journal of the American Thyroid Association. 2000;**10**:573-577

[36] Sherman SI, Tielens ET, Sostre S, Wharam MD Jr, Ladenson PW. Clinical utility of posttreatment radioiodine scans in the management of patients with thyroid carcinoma. The Journal of clinical endocrinology and metabolism. 1994;**78**:629-634

[37] Haugen BR, Alexander EK, Bible KC, Doherty GM, Mandel SJ, et al. 2015 American Thyroid Association Management Guidelines for Adult Patients with Thyroid Nodules and Differentiated Thyroid Cancer: The American Thyroid Association Guidelines Task Force on Thyroid Nodules and Differentiated Thyroid Cancer. Thyroid. 2016;**26**:1-133

[38] Saracyn M, Bilski M, Kamiński G, Niemczyk S. Can radioiodine be administered effectively and safely to a patient with severe chronic kidney disease? Clinical Endocrinology. 2014;**81**:169-174

[39] Yeyin N, Cavdar I, Uslu L, Abuqbeitah M, Demir M. Effects of hemodialysis on iodine-131 biokinetics in thyroid carcinoma patients with end- stage chronic renal failure. Nuclear Medicine Communications. 2016;**37**:283-287

[40] Ruel E, Thomas S, Dinan M, Perkins JM, Roman SA, Sosa JA. Adjuvant radioactive iodine therapy is associated with improved survival for patients with intermediate-risk papillary thyroid cancer. The Journal of Clinical Endocrinology and Metabolism. 2015;**100**:1529-1536

[41] Kazaure HS, Roman SA, Sosa JA. Aggressive variants of papillary thyroid cancer: Incidence, characteristics and predictors of survival among 43,738 patients. Annals of Surgical Oncology. 2012;**19**:1874-1880

[42] Kazaure HS, Roman SA, Sosa JA. Insular thyroid cancer: A population-level analysis of patient characteristics and predictors of survival. Cancer. 2012;**118**:3260-3267

[43] Liu J, Liu Y, Lin Y, Liang J. Radioactive iodine-refractory differentiated thyroid cancer and redifferentiation therapy. Endocrinology Metabolism (Seoul). 2019 Sep;**34**(3):215-225

[44] Kirtane K, Roth MY. Emerging therapies for radioactive iodine refractory thyroid cancer. Current Treatment Options in Oncology. 2020;**21**(3):18

[45] Knauf JA, Sartor MA, Medvedovic M, Lundsmith E, Ryder M, Salzano M, et al. Progression of BRAF-induced thyroid cancer is associated with epithelial-mesenchymal transition requiring concomitant MAP kinase and TGFβ signaling. Oncogene. 2011;**30**(28):3153-3162

[46] Hu S, Liu D, Tufano RP, Carson KA, Rosenbaum E, Cohen Y, et al. Association of aberrant methylation of tumor suppres- sor genes with tumor aggressiveness and BRAF mutation in papillary thyroid cancer. International Journal of Cancer. 2006;**119**:2322-2329

[47] Trapasso F, Iuliano R, Chiefari E, Arturi F, Stella A, Filetti S, et al. Iodide sym. porter gene expression in normal and transformed rat thyroid cells. European Journal of Endocrinology. 1999;**140**:447-451

[48] Wang J, Knauf JA, Basu S, Puxeddu E, Kuroda H, Santoro M, et al. Conditional expression of RET/PTC induces a weak oncogenic drive in thyroid PCCL3 cells and inhibits thyrotropin action at multiple levels. Molecular Endocrinology. 2003;**17**:1425-1436

[49] Schmidbauer B, Menhart K, Hellwig D, Grosse J. Differentiated thyroid cancer-treatment: State of the art. International Journal of Molecular Sciences. 2017;**18**:1292

[50] Luster M, Clarke SE, Dietlein M, Lassmann M, Lind P, et al. European Association of Nuclear Medicine (EANM). Guidelines for radioiodine therapy of differentiated thyroid cancer. European Journal of Nuclear Medicine and Molecular Imaging. 2008;**35**:1941-1959

[51] Tiedje V, Schmid KW, Weber F, Bockisch A, Führer D. Differenzierte Schilddrüsenkarzinome. Internist (Berl). 2015;**56**:153-166

[52] Pacini F, Schlumberger M, Dralle H, Elisei R, Smit JW, et al. European Thyroid Cancer Taskforce. European consensus for the management of patients with differentiated thyroid carcinoma of the follicular epithelium. European Journal of Endocrinology. 2006;**154**:787-803

[53] Piccardo A, Trimboli P, Foppiani L, Treglia G, Ferrarazzo G, et al. PET/CT in thyroid nodule and differentiated thyroid cancer patients. The evidence-based state of the art. Reviews in Endocrine & Metabolic Disorders. 2019;**20**:47-64

Chapter 7

Systemic Therapy in Thyroid Cancer

Geethu Babu, Rejnish Ravikumar, Malu Rafi, Lekha Madhavan Nair, Zuzaki Sharafuddin, John Mathew, Nijo Jose and Kainickal Cessal Thommachan

Abstract

The standard treatment for patients with differentiated thyroid cancer (DTC) is a combination of surgery, radioactive iodine (RAI), and long-term thyroid hormone–suppression therapy. Treatment of patients whose diseases persist, recur, or metastasize remains a challenge. The role of cytotoxic chemotherapy in the treatment of thyroid cancer is limited. The key signaling pathways involved in the pathogenesis of thyroid cancers are the RAS/RAF/MEK & PI3K/Akt/mTOR pathways. Systemic therapy in thyroid cancer involves the use of tyrosine kinase inhibitors targeting the above mentioned pathways which are often both effective in controlling disease and have manageable toxicity. Sorafenib and lenvatinib are approved for advanced radioiodine refractory and poorly differentiated thyroid cancers and vandetanib and cabozantinib for recurrent or metastatic medullary thyroid cancers. Cabozantinib is also approved for the treatment of locally advanced or metastatic radioactive iodine–refractory differentiated thyroid cancer that has progressed after prior VEGF-targeted therapy. The combination of dabrafenib (BRAF inhibitor) and trametinib (MEK inhibitor) is approved for BRAF V600E mutated unresectable locally advanced anaplastic thyroid cancer. Selpercatinib, RET kinase inhibitor is used for advanced and metastatic RET mutated medullary thyroid cancers and advanced and metastatic RET fusion-positive thyroid cancers of any histologic type. Various clinical trials using newer molecules targeting the aforementioned pathways are ongoing.

Keywords: carcinoma thyroid, Iodine refractory, tyrosine kinase inhibitors, anaplastic and medullary thyroid cancer, differentiated thyroid cancer (DTC)

1. Introduction

The incidence of thyroid cancers is on the rise with over 586,202 new patients diagnosed and greater than 43,646 deaths recorded each year worldwide [1]. Thyroid cancers arise from either of the two cell types, namely follicular and parafollicular cells. Differentiated thyroid cancer (DTC) accounts for 95% of all thyroid cancers [2] and has three subtypes, papillary thyroid cancer (PTC), follicular thyroid cancer

(FTC), and Hurthle cell thyroid cancer (HCTC). The poorly differentiated or undifferentiated category includes anaplastic thyroid cancer (ATC). Differentiated and undifferentiated tumors originate in follicular cells and medullary thyroid cancer (MTC) arises from parafollicular or C cells. While surgery remains the mainstay of the treatment of all different histologies of thyroid cancers, for differentiated thyroid cancers, radioactive iodine and TSH suppression therapy also play an important role in adjuvant management [3]. The prognosis of thyroid cancer, with the exception of anaplastic thyroid cancer is excellent with the standard therapy. Treatment of patients whose diseases persist, recur, or metastasize remains challenging. Cytotoxic chemotherapy has limited role in the treatment of thyroid cancer, hence there was an urgent need for the development of new more effective therapies for that subset of patients. Recent developments in understanding the molecular etiologies of thyroid cancer have led to the identification of novel precision oncological treatments that are significantly improving the outlook for patients with advanced diseases and a new era of treatment options emerged. Targeted therapy with kinase inhibitors has shown promise in management of metastatic and recurrent thyroid cancer. This chapter summarizes the rationale for using systemic therapy and the approved drugs in recurrent or metastatic thyroid carcinoma.

2. Molecular pathogenesis of thyroid cancer

Thyroid cancers arise as a result of the accumulation of multiple genetic mutations that cause abnormal cellular proliferation and prolonged survival of malignant cells. Most thyroid cancers arise as a result of aberrant signaling involving the PI3K/Akt/mTOR and MAPK signaling pathways. The PI3K and MAPK pathways are activated by receptor tyrosine kinase (RTK). The PI3K/Akt/mTOR pathway is classically activated by the induction of RTK at the cell membrane. Activated intracellular PI3K then phosphorylates and activates AKT. AKT then travels inside the nucleus to upregulate various other oncogenes as well the mTOR pathway, that later trigger tumorigenesis. MAPK signaling is stimulated first by activation of an RTK similar to the PI3K/Akt/mTOR pathway. RTK then activates multiple other genes, including MEK, ERK, RAS, and BRAF. ERK ultimately enters the nucleus and then promotes tumorigenesis. The most common of genetic changes in Papillary Thyroid Cancers are point mutations in *BRAF* (40%) [4] and *RAS* (38%) genes [5]. Rearrangement of the *RET/PTC* proto-oncogene occurs in ~10–20% of papillary cancers [6]. Genetic rearrangements and mutations in anaplastic lymphoma kinase (*ALK*) [7] and neurotrophic tropomyosin receptor kinase *(NTRK)1-3* are also present [8], but only ~1–2% of cases. Point mutations of *RAS* and rearrangements of *PPARγ/PAX8* genes are the most common oncogenic alteration in follicular thyroid cancers. Mutations in members of the PI3K pathway, such as *PTEN* deletion/mutation and *PIK3CA*, have also been reported at low frequencies [9]. Both Anaplastic and Poorly Differentiated Thyroid Cancers also demonstrate a high prevalence of the *TP53* and *TERT* promoter mutations, which is usually associated with greater aggressiveness [10]. The most common genetic alterations found in Medullary Thyroid Cancer cells are the *RET*-activating point mutations [11], whereas *RAS* mutations, mainly the *HRAS* and *KRAS* mutations, have been reported in ~17%of cases [12].

Angiogenesis, being a very important process in tumor development is another attractive target for cancer therapy [9]. The vascular endothelial growth factor (VEGF) is overexpressed in the setting of intratumoral hypoxia via hypoxia-inducible factor-1α (HIF1α) and promotes angiogenesis. This transcription factor HIF1α is also upregulated by MAPK and PI3K/AKT pathways. An important target of HIF1α is the MET receptor, which is highly expressed in many thyroid cancers, promoting angiogenesis, cellular motility, invasion, and metastasis [13]. The above mentioned molecular pathways have been the basis for development of newer drugs and their testing in clinical trials in recent years and thereby provide attractive therapeutic targets for thyroid cancer.

3. Systemic therapy in thyroid cancer

3.1 Chemotherapeutic agents

Cytotoxic chemotherapy has limited role in treatment of thyroid cancer, as most trials using cytotoxic chemotherapies in thyroid cancer have shown disappointing efficacy. FDA approved doxorubicin for the treatment of thyroid cancer in 1974. Chemotherapy regimens with doxorubicin have shown 30–45% partial response in differentiated thyroid cancers [14, 15]. The combination of cisplatin and doxorubicin did not result in any additional improvement in overall response compared to doxorubicin alone [16]. Various other combination chemotherapy regimens also have not yielded any encouraging results so far [17, 18]. Chemotherapy is generally not recommended for patients with differentiated thyroid cancers in view of poor response rates, short duration of response, and toxic effects of chemotherapy [19]. Similar to DTC, chemotherapy has a limited role in the treatment of persistent or recurrent MTC due to the poor response rates (10–15% partial response) [20]. Combination chemotherapy regimens based on dacarbazine and doxorubicin have been tried in MTC, but with limited results [21]. In anaplastic thyroid cancers, chemotherapy in addition to surgery and radiation showed longer median survival rates for stage IVA and IVC ATC patients in a US national cancer registry study [22]. Few other studies have also demonstrated the utility of neoadjuvant chemotherapy in patients with stage IVA and IVB tumors allowing them to undergo successful resection [23]. In advanced cases, doxorubicin, taxanes (paclitaxel or docetaxel) and platins (cisplatin or carboplatin) have demonstrated activity with response rates ranging from 15 to 25% [24, 25].

3.2 Targeted therapies

Evolution of targeted therapies in thyroid cancer:

The increasing knowledge about the molecular alterations underlying thyroid cancer has greatly increased the interest in developing new drugs for targeted treatments in the last decade. The families of drugs that have primarily been investigated and most extensively studied for the treatment of thyroid cancer are tyrosine kinase inhibitors (TKIs). The first international clinical trial started in 2005 and explored the efficacy of motesanib diphosphate on 93 patients with progressive, locally advanced or metastatic, radioiodine refractory DTC. The median PFS was estimated to be 40 weeks [26]. The same drug was investigated for the treatment of locally advanced or metastatic, progressive, or symptomatic MTC in another single-arm phase 2 study which enrolled 91 patients. The median PFS was 48 weeks [27]. Despite these promising results, the drug was not FDA approved for these indications. Both studies used a single-arm design and were performed in a relatively small population of patients. Moreover, the lack of a placebo arm is another limitation. Soon after the motesanib study, another, phase 2 study examining the effect of axitinib on 52 cases of locally advanced, unresectable, or metastatic MTC or RAI-R DTC was started. The median PFS and OS was 16.1 months and 27.2 months respectively. As in the previous studies, the single-arm design of this study makes the interpretation of the results rather difficult. Although the results appeared encouraging, no further studies have been planned using this drug [28]. These trials show that targeted therapies could lead to prolonged disease stabilization and objective response in patients with metastatic or recurrent thyroid cancers. Following these multiple other targeted agents soon entered clinical trials and there by a new era of treatment options emerged.

3.2.1 Multikinase inhibitors

Various multikinase inhibitors has proven to be an effective treatment option for metastatic and recurrent Thyroid Cancers, given the activity of the PI3K/Akt/mTOR and MAPK signaling pathways in this disease. Currently, there are four drugs, all oral multikinase inhibitors, approved in the treatment of differentiated and medullary thyroid cancer. Sorafenib is a multikinase inhibitor that targets the VEGF receptor (VEGFR), platelet-derived growth factor receptor (PDGFR), and RAF. Lenvatinib is another kinase inhibitor that targets VEGFR1–3, fibroblast growth factor receptors (FGFR) 1–4, PDGFRα, RET, and c-Kit signaling pathways. Vandetanib selectively targets RET, VEGFR, and EGFR signaling and cabozantinib is a kinase inhibitor of RET, VEGFR2, and MET. All these kinase inhibitors are antiangiogenic, but they also have additional targets that may contribute to their efficacy. The response rates of the above agents vary from 30 to 50% in various trials.

Sorafenib and lenvatinib are FDA approved for advanced radioiodine refractory and poorly differentiated thyroid cancers and vandetanib and cabozantinib are approved for recurrent or metastatic medullary thyroid cancers.

Role of multikinase inhibitors in differentiated thyroid cancer:

Two randomized placebo-controlled phase III clinical trials that led to US Food and Drug Administration (FDA) approval of TKIs for treatment of progressive RAI-refractory DTC are the DECISION and SELECT trials.

Sorafenib was approved by the FDA in 2013 on the basis of DECISION trial in locally advanced or metastatic radioiodine refractory differentiated thyroid cancer [29]. DECISION, a double-blind, placebo-controlled, phase 3 trial trial reported a significant progression-free survival (PFS) benefit of 5 months with sorafenib. Median progression-free survival in the sorafenib group was 10·8 months vs. 5·8 months in the placebo group ($p < 0{\cdot}0001$). However, the overall response rate [ORR] was 12% in the trial. Sorafenib did not improve overall survival (OS), although PFS was longer with sorafenib. The SELECT trial, a phase 3 randomized double-blind trial investigated lenvatinib versus placebo in patients with progressive iodine-refractory DTC which showed a significant improvement in PFS of 14 months with lenvatinib compared with placebo. The median PFS was 18.3 months in the lenvatinib group and 3.6 months in the placebo group ($P < 0.001$) and lenvatinib had an ORR of 65% [30].

Cabozantinib has shown activity in patients with radioiodine-refractory DTC who have been previously treated with lenvatinib, sorafenib, or both TKIs in COSMIC -311, a double-blind, placebo-controlled, phase 3 trial [31]. The trial showed significant improvement in progression-free survival for cabozantinib over placebo (5·7 versus 1·9 months, $p < 0{\cdot}0001$) and an ORR of 15%.Based on the above trial results, FDA approved cabozantinib for the treatment of locally advanced or metastatic radioactive iodine–refractory differentiated thyroid cancer that has progressed after prior VEGF-targeted therapy in 2021.

Role of multikinase inhibitors in medullary thyroid cancer:

Vandetanib was approved for the treatment of locally advanced or metastatic medullary thyroid cancer based on the ZETA trial, a randomized double blind phase 3 trial that demonstrated a PFS benefit of 11 months (p < 0.0001) with vandetanib compared with placebo in patients with MTC. At a median follow up of 24 months, vandetanib demonstrated an ORR of 45% [32]. One major limitation in the design of the study was that there was no requirement for disease progression prior to enrolment in the trial. Because of the above limitation, patients with indolent disease could have been part of this clinical trial.

In the EXAM trial a double-blind, phase III trial, which investigated cabozantinib versus placebo in locally advanced or metastatic medullary thyroid cancer, patients were required to have disease progression at the time of study entry. At a median follow-up of 13.9 months, the trial showed that the placebo arm had a much shorter PFS of 4 months compared with 11 months for those in the cabozantinib arm (p < .001), with an ORR of 28% [33]. The below table summarises the four approved kinase inhibitors used in thyroid cancers (**Table 1**).

Drug	**Sorafenib (DECISION TRIAL) [29]**	**Lenvatinib (SELECT trial) [30]**	**Vandetanib (ZETA trial) [32]**	**Cabozantinib (EXAM trial) [33]**	**Cabozantinib (COSMIC trial) [31]**
Tumor	DTC -Radioiodine refractory	DTC -Radioiodine refractory	Medullary Thyroid cancer	Medullary Thyroid cancer	DTC -Radioiodine refractory progressing following VEGFR targeted therapy
Targets	VEGFR,c-Kit, RET, PDGFR, RAS	VEGFR,c-Kit, RET, PDGFR, FGFR	VEGFR,c-Kit, RET, EGFR	VEGFR,c-Kit, RET, ERT, MET	VEGFR,c-Kit, RET, ERT, MET
No of patients	417	392	331	330	187
PR%	12.2%	64.8%	45%	28%	15%
Median PFS (Months)	10.8	18.3	30.5	11.3	5.7
Side effects	Palmer-plantar erythro dysesthesia, Diarrhea, alopecia,skin rash, fatigue, weight loss, anorexia, hypertension	Hypertension, Fatigue, Diarrhea, Anorexia, Weight loss, Nausea, Stomatitis	Diarrhea, Skin rash, Nausea, Hypertension Qt-prolongation	Diarrhea, Palmer-plantar erythro dysesthesia, weight loss, anorexia, Nausea, Fatigue, Gi ulcers & hemorrhage	Diarrhea, Palmer-plantar erythro dysesthesia, weight loss, anorexia, Nausea, Fatigue, Gi ulcers & hemorrhage

Table 1.
Four approved kinase inhibitors based on their phase 3outcomes.

3.2.2 Selective inhibitors

3.2.2.1 BRAF and/or MEK inhibitors

Role of BRAF and/or MEK inhibitors in Anaplastic thyroid cancer:

BRAF inhibitors alone, or in combination with MEK inhibitors, have been extensively studied in *BRAF* mutated thyroid cancer. Dabrafenib (BRAF inhibitor) and trametinib (MEK1/2inhibitor) was FDA approved for BRAFV600E mutated ATC based on the safety and efficacy data in a phase II, open-label BRF117019 trial in which 16 patients with BRAF V600E mutant ATC were enrolled [34]. At a median follow-up of 47 weeks, the ORR was 69%. Seven of the 16 patients had continued response to therapy. Median overall survival and progression free survival were not reached in the study. The common adverse effects observed in the study were fatigue, pyrexia, and nausea.

The outcomes of a series of six initially unresectable *BRAF* V600E mutated ATC patients who received neoadjuvant dabrafenib and trametinib followed by a R1 or R0 surgical resection was reported by Wang et al. All six patients continued treatment with dabrafenib and trametinib after surgery. All six patients could undergo complete surgical resection. Analysis of the surgical specimen revealed 0–5% viability in five patients, whereas it was 50% viable in one patient. OS at 6 months and 1 year was 100% and 83%, respectively and loco-regional control rate was 100% in the series [35]. In a large single-institution cohort study at MD Anderson Cancer Center on 479 patients with ATC treated from 2000 to 2019, there were 20 patients treated with BRAF directed neoadjuvant targeted therapy followed by surgery. The 1-year overall survival was 94% in this group [36].

Role of BRAF and/or MEK inhibitors in differentiated thyroid cancer:

BRAF inhibitiors (vemurafenib or dabrafenib) alone or in combination with MEK inhibitors are effective for differentiated thyroid cancers. Vemurafenib was tested in 51 patients with BRAF V600E mutated PTC in a non-randomized, open-label phase II study. 10 of 26 patients who were VEGFR tyrosine kinase inhibitor-naive had partial response (PR) rates of 38.5%, and a majority had at least stable disease (SD) (57.5%). Median PFS was 18.2 months and Median OS was not reached [37]. In another phase II, randomized study, patients with BRAFV600E mutated PTC were randomized to dabrafenib monotherapy or dabrafenib with trametinib. 10 of 26 patients, who received dabrafenib monotherapy, had RECIST defined partial response, while nine of 27 in the combination arm had a partial response of the disease. A total of 50% and 54% in monotherapy and combination, respectively, had at least 20% decrease in target lesions. Median PFS for dabrafinib and trametinib combination was 15.1 months vs. 11.4 months for dabrafenib alone [38].

Mammalian target of rapamycin (mTOR) inhibitors:

The PI3K/Akt/mTOR pathway is downstream of RAS and activation of this pathway mostly occurs in advanced thyroid cancers. Everolimus and temsirolimus are drugs that are inhibitors of the mTOR pathway. These drugs have been studied in several phase 2 clinical trials of all thyroid cancer subtypes.

50 patients (33 DTC, including 13 HCTC; 10 MTC; and 7 ATC) were enrolled in the most recently published everolimus trial by Hanna *et al.* Disease progression within previous 6 months was an inclusion criterion for enrollment to the trial. Six percent of patients in the trial achieved partial response and 74% of patients experienced stable disease. The median PFS was 12.5 months for the entire cohort of patients in the trial. The median PFS in DTC and MTC was 12.9 and 13.1 months, respectively [39].

The combination of everolimus with other targeted agents has also been tried. In a trial combining everolimus and sorafenib, 55% of patients achieved partial response, which is higher than single-agent sorafenib reported in literature [40].

Similarly, when a combination of sorafenib and temsirolimus was studied in follicular-derived thyroid cancer, partial response was seen in 22% patients [10]. Adverse effects of m-TOR inhibitors include mucositis, anorexia, pancytopenia, hyperglycemia, liver function test abnormalities, and rarely pneumonitis.

3.2.2.2 Selective RET inhibitors

Selpercatinib is an oral selective RET kinase inhibitor for RET mutated MTC and RET fusion-positive thyroid cancers. The safety and efficacy of selpercatinib (160 mg twice daily) in patients with RET-mutant MTC was evaluated in the phase I/II LIBRETTO-001 trial. The ORR was 69% among 55 patients previously treated with TKIs including cabozantinib and vandetinib. Among 88 TKI naïve subjects, ORR was 73% and ORR was 62% in a cohort of patients with RET-fusion positive thyroid cancer [41]. Selpercatinib is well tolerated with very few adverse effects reported like fatigue, diarrhea, constipation, dry mouth, nausea, and dyspnea. Pralsetinib, is a second potent RET-inhibitor with activity in RET-fusion positive MTC. ARROW is a phase I/II trial of pralsetinib for RET-mutated cancers. Among 13 RET- fusion positive thyroid cancer patients enrolled in the trial, overall response rates were 91% and all patients had at least stable disease. For RET-mutated treatment naïve MTC patients, overall response rates were 74%, while overall response rates of around 60% were reported for previously treated patients [42]. Pralsetinib is also well tolerated like selpercatinib, with constipation, elevated liver enzymes, hypertension, fatigue, and peripheral oedema being the most common side effects.

3.2.2.3 Other selective inhibitors

The existence of gene fusions in *NTRK*, *ALK*, and *ROS1* in a subgroup of patients with PTC, PDTC, and ATC has added to the understanding of the genetic basis of thyroid cancer and such patients may have more aggressive disease. Larotrectinib is a selective pan-NTRK (A, B, and C) inhibitor. Larotrectinib has been studied in cancer patients that harbor NTRK fusions, including in those with NTRK fusion–positive DTC and ATC [43]. In a study of 28 patients with TRK fusion–positive iodine-refractory DTC, ORR was 75% [44]. Overall, larotrectinib was well tolerated and the most common adverse effects reported were fatigue, nausea, vomiting, abnormal liver function tests and dizziness.

Entrectinib is a potent inhibitor of NTRK like larotrectinib, but it also targets ROS1 and ALK [45]. NCT02568267, an open-label, multicenter, global, phase 2 basket study of entrectinib is enrolling patients with thyroid tumors (including PTC) harboring gene rearrangements in *NTRK*, *ROS1*, or *ALK*.

There is one case report reported in literature of an ATC patient with an *ALK* rearrangement, who has been successfully treated with crizotinib (an ALK inhibitor) after failing standard therapy [46]. An open-label study of ceritinib, an ALK inhibitor, recruiting ATC patients (NCT02289144) is currently ongoing.

3.3 Immunotherapy

Immuno-oncology is another area that is gaining momentum in advanced thyroid cancer, including immune checkpoint blockade. Inhibition of programmed cell death

Study number	Treatments	Thyroid cancer type	Status
NCT04400474 [47]	Cabozantinib with Atezolizumab	ATC	Phase II, Recruiting
NCT04238624 [48]	Cemiplimab with Dabrafenib and Trametinib	ATC	Phase II, Recruiting
NCT03360890 [49]	Pembrolizumab and Chemotherapy	ATC	Phase II, Recruiting
NCT04171622 [50]	Lenvatinib and Pembrolizumab	ATC	Phase II, Not yet recruiting
NCT03181100 [51]	Atezolizumab with Chemotherapy	ATC/PDTC	Phase II, Recruiting
NCT03914300 [52]	Cabozantinib, Nivolumab, and Ipilimumab	Advanced DTC	Phase II, Suspended (scheduled interim monitoring)
NCT04061980 [53]	Encorafenib and Binimetinib and/or Nivolumab	BRAF V600Epositive DTC	Phase II, Recruiting
NCT04675710 [54]	Pembrolizumab, Dabrafenib, and Trametinib	ATC, PDTC	Phase II, Recruiting
NCT02973997 [55]	Lenvatinib and Pembrolizumab	DTC, PDTC	Phase II, Active, Not recruiting
NCT04731740 [56]	Pembrolizumab and Lenvatinib or Chemotherapy	PDTC, ATC	Phase II, Suspended (Financial problems)
NCT03246958 [57]	Nivolumab and Ipilimumab	DTC, MTC, ATC	Phase II, Active, Not recruiting
NCT04524884 [58]	Toripalimab and Surufatinib	MTC, DTC	Phase II, Not yet recruiting
NCT04521348 [59]	Camrelizumab and Famitinib	MTC, ATC, DTC	Phase II, Recruiting
NCT03753919 [60]	Durvalumab with Tremelimumab	ATC, DTC, MTC	Phase II, Recruiting

Table 2.
Ongoing clinical trials of immuno-oncology treatments for thyroid cancer.

protein (PD-1), cytotoxic T-lymphocyte-associated protein 4 (CTLA-4) and other proteins in the checkpoint cascade, is currently being investigated as new molecular targets in patients with advanced thyroid cancers (**Table 2**). Updated guidelines that incorporate testing for immuno-oncology markers may need to be developed depending on the results of these trials.

4. Conclusions

Recent understanding on the molecular basis of thyroid cancers have led to newer advances in treatment approaches for patients with advanced and recurrent disease. Patients with advanced radioiodine refractory DTC, PDTC were considered to have poor prognoses until recently. The role of cytotoxic chemotherapy in treatment of thyroid cancer is limited. Sorafenib and lenvatinib are approved for advanced radioiodine refractory and poorly differentiated thyroid cancers and vandetanib and cabozantinib for recurrent or metastatic medullary thyroid cancers. Cabozantinib is also approved for the treatment of locally advanced or metastatic radioactive iodine–refractory differentiated thyroid cancer that has progressed after prior VEGF-targeted therapy. The combination of the BRAF inhibitor, dabrafenib and MEK inhibitor, trametinib, is approved for *BRAF* V600E mutated; unresectable locally advanced anaplastic thyroid cancer. Selpercatinib, RET kinase inhibitor is used for advanced RET mutated medullary thyroid cancers and RET fusion-positive thyroid cancers of any histologic type. Due to the availability of drugs that target specific molecular alterations for the treatment of thyroid cancers, optimal molecular testing to identify suitable candidates for such therapies is warranted. The knowledge of the molecular profile of the tumor allows informed treatment decisions to be made, though optimal therapeutic sequencing of targeted therapy or their combination with immunotherapy is not yet known. More data from ongoing clinical trials might help to document the optimal therapeutic sequencing of available molecular therapies.

Author details

Geethu Babu, Rejnish Ravikumar, Malu Rafi, Lekha Madhavan Nair, Zuzaki Sharafuddin, John Mathew, Nijo Jose and Kainickal Cessal Thommachan*
Department of Radiation Oncology, Regional Cancer Centre, Thiruvananthapuram, Kerala, India

*Address all correspondence to: drcessalthomas@gmail.com

References

[1] Sung H, Ferlay J, Siegel RL, Laversanne M, Soerjomataram I, Jemal A, et al. Global cancer statistics 2020: GLOBOCAN estimates of incidence and mortality worldwide for 36 cancers in 185 countries. CA: A Cancer Journal for Clinicians. 2021;**71**(3):209-249

[2] Haugen BR, Alexander EK, Bible KC, Doherty GM, Mandel SJ, Nikiforov YE, et al. 2015 american thyroid association management guidelines for adult patients with thyroid nodules and differentiated thyroid cancer: The American thyroid association guidelines task force on thyroid nodules and differentiated thyroid cancer. Thyroid. 2016;**26**(1):1-133

[3] Cabanillas ME, McFadden DG, Durante C. Thyroid cancer. Lancet. 2016;**388**(10061):2783-2795

[4] Cohen Y, Xing M, Mambo E, Guo Z, Wu G, Trink B, et al. BRAF mutation in papillary thyroid carcinoma. JNCI. 2003;**95**(8):625-627

[5] Kimura ET, Nikiforova MN, Zhu Z, Knauf JA, Nikiforov YE, Fagin JA. High prevalence of BRAF mutations in thyroid cancer: genetic evidence for constitutive activation of the RET/PTC-RAS-BRAF signaling pathway in papillary thyroid carcinoma1. Cancer Research. 2003;**63**(7):1454-1457

[6] Grieco M, Santoro M, Berlingieri MT, Melillo RM, Donghi R, Bongarzone I, et al. PTC is a novel rearranged form of the ret proto-oncogene and is frequently detected in vivo in human thyroid papillary carcinomas. Cell. 1990;**60**(4):557-563

[7] Chou A, Fraser S, Toon CW, Clarkson A, Sioson L, Farzin M, et al. A detailed clinicopathologic study of ALK-translocated papillary thyroid carcinoma. The American Journal of Surgical Pathology. 2015;**39**(5):652-659

[8] Pierotti MA, Bongarzone I, Borrello MG, Mariani C, Miranda C, Sozzi G, et al. Rearrangements of TRK proto-oncogene in papillary thyroid carcinomas. Journal of Endocrinological Investigation. 1995;**18**(2):130-133

[9] Xing M. Molecular pathogenesis and mechanisms of thyroid cancer. Nature Reviews Cancer. 2013 Mar; **13**(3):184-199

[10] Landa I, Ibrahimpasic T, Boucai L, Sinha R, Knauf JA, Shah RH, et al. Genomic and transcriptomic hallmarks of poorly differentiated and anaplastic thyroid cancers. The Journal of Clinical Investigation. 2016;**126**(3):1052-1066

[11] Romei C, Casella F, Tacito A, Bottici V, Valerio L, Viola D, et al. New insights in the molecular signature of advanced medullary thyroid cancer: Evidence of a bad outcome of cases with double RET mutations. Journal of Medical Genetics. 2016;**53**(11):729-734

[12] Ciampi R, Mian C, Fugazzola L, Cosci B, Romei C, Barollo S, et al. Evidence of a low prevalence of RAS mutations in a large medullary thyroid cancer series. Thyroid. 2013;**23**(1):50-57

[13] Scarpino S, Cancellario d'Alena F, Di Napoli A, Pasquini A, Marzullo A, Ruco LP. Increased expression of Met protein is associated with up-regulation of hypoxia inducible factor-1 (HIF-1) in tumour cells in papillary carcinoma of the thyroid. The Journal of Pathology. 2004;**202**(3):352-358

[14] Gottlieb JA, Hill CS. Chemotherapy of thyroid cancer with adriamycin. Experience with 30 patients. The New England Journal of Medicine. 1974;**290**(4):193-197

[15] Droz JP, Schlumberger M, Rougier P, Ghosn M, Gardet P, Parmentier C. Chemotherapy in metastatic nonanaplastic thyroid cancer: experience at the Institut Gustave-Roussy. Tumori. 1990;**76**(5):480-483

[16] Shimaoka K, Schoenfeld DA, Dewys WD, Creech RH, Deconti R. A randomized trial of doxorubicin versus doxorubicin plus cisplatin in patients with advanced thyroid carcinoma. Cancer. 1985;**56**(9):2155-2160

[17] Spano JP, Vano Y, Vignot S, De La Motte RT, Hassani L, Mouawad R, et al. GEMOX regimen in the treatment of metastatic differentiated refractory thyroid carcinoma. Medical Oncology. 2012;**29**(3):1421-1428

[18] Argiris A, Agarwala SS, Karamouzis MV, Burmeister LA, Carty SE. A phase II trial of doxorubicin and interferon alpha 2b in advanced, non-medullary thyroid cancer. Investigational New Drugs. 2008;**26**(2):183-188

[19] Sherman SI. Cytotoxic chemotherapy for differentiated thyroid carcinoma. Clinical Oncology. 2010;**22**(6):464-468

[20] Orlandi F, Caraci P, Berruti A, Puligheddu B, Pivano G, Dogliotti L, et al. Chemotherapy with dacarbazine and 5-fluorouracil in advanced medullary thyroid cancer. Annals of Oncology. 1994;**5**(8):763-765

[21] Petursson SR. Metastatic medullary thyroid carcinoma. Complete response to combination chemotherapy with dacarbazine and 5-fluorouracil. Cancer. 1988;**62**(9):1899-1903

[22] Haymart MR, Banerjee M, Yin H, Worden F, Griggs JJ. Marginal treatment benefit in anaplastic thyroid cancer. Cancer. 2013;**119**(17):3133-3139

[23] Higashiyama T, Ito Y, Hirokawa M, Fukushima M, Uruno T, Miya A, et al. Induction chemotherapy with weekly paclitaxel administration for anaplastic thyroid carcinoma. Thyroid. 2010;**20**(1):7-14

[24] Kawada K, Kitagawa K, Kamei S, Inada M, Mitsuma A, Sawaki M, et al. The feasibility study of docetaxel in patients with anaplastic thyroid cancer. Japanese Journal of Clinical Oncology. 2010;**40**(6):596-599

[25] Ain KB, Egorin MJ, DeSimone PA. Treatment of anaplastic thyroid carcinoma with paclitaxel: Phase 2 trial using ninety-six-hour infusion. Thyroid. 2000;**10**(7):587-594

[26] Sherman SI, Wirth LJ, Droz JP, Hofmann M, Bastholt L, Martins RG, et al. Motesanib Thyroid Cancer Study Group. Motesanib diphosphate in progressive differentiated thyroid cancer. The New England Journal of Medicine. 2008 Jul 3;**359**(1):31-42. DOI: 10.1056/NEJMoa075853. PMID: 18596272

[27] Schlumberger MJ, Elisei R, Bastholt L, Wirth LJ, Martins RG, Locati LD, et al. Phase II study of safety and efficacy of motesanib in patients with progressive or symptomatic, advanced or metastatic medullary thyroid cancer. Journal of Clinical Oncology. 2009;**27**(23):3794-3801

[28] Locati LD, Licitra L, Agate L, Ou SHI, Boucher A, Jarzab B, et al. Treatment of advanced thyroid cancer with axitinib: Phase 2 study with pharmacokinetic/pharmacodynamic and quality-of-life assessments. Cancer. 2014;**120**(17):2694-2703

[29] Brose MS, Nutting CM, Jarzab B, Elisei R, Siena S, Bastholt L, et al. Sorafenib in radioactive iodine-refractory, locally advanced or metastatic differentiated thyroid cancer: a randomised, double-blind, phase 3 trial. Lancet. 2014;**384**(9940):319-328

[30] Schlumberger M, Tahara M, Wirth LJ, Robinson B, Brose MS, Elisei R, et al. Lenvatinib versus placebo in radioiodine-refractory thyroid cancer. The New England Journal of Medicine. 2015;**372**(7):621-630

[31] Brose MS, Robinson B, Sherman SI, Krajewska J, Lin CC, Vaisman F, et al. Cabozantinib for radioiodine-refractory differentiated thyroid cancer (COSMIC-311): A randomised, double-blind, placebo-controlled, phase 3 trial. The Lancet Oncology. 2021;**22**(8):1126-1138

[32] Wells SA, Robinson BG, Gagel RF, Dralle H, Fagin JA, Santoro M, et al. Vandetanib in patients with locally advanced or metastatic medullary thyroid cancer: A randomized, double-blind phase III trial. Journal of Clinical Oncology: Official Journal of the American Society of Clinical Oncology. 2012;**30**(2):134-141

[33] Elisei R, Schlumberger MJ, Müller SP, Schöffski P, Brose MS, Shah MH, et al. Cabozantinib in progressive medullary thyroid cancer. Journal of Clinical Oncology: Official Journal of the American Society of Clinical Oncology. 2013;**31**(29):3639-3646

[34] Subbiah V, Kreitman RJ, Wainberg ZA, Cho JY, Schellens JHM, Soria JC, et al. Dabrafenib and trametinib treatment in patients with locally advanced or metastatic BRAF V600-mutant anaplastic thyroid cancer. Journal of Clinical Oncology: Official Journal of the American Society of Clinical Oncology. 2018;**36**(1):7-13

[35] Wang JR, Zafereo ME, Dadu R, Ferrarotto R, Busaidy NL, Lu C, et al. Complete surgical resection following neoadjuvant dabrafenib plus trametinib in BRAFV600E-mutated anaplastic thyroid carcinoma. Thyroid. 2019;**29**(8):1036-1043

[36] Maniakas A, Dadu R, Busaidy NL, Wang JR, Ferrarotto R, Lu C, et al. Evaluation of overall survival in patients with anaplastic thyroid carcinoma, 2000-2019. JAMA Oncology. 2020;**6**(9):1397-1404

[37] Brose MS, Cabanillas ME, Cohen EEW, Wirth LJ, Riehl T, Yue H, et al. Vemurafenib in patients with BRAF(V600E)-positive metastatic or unresectable papillary thyroid cancer refractory to radioactive iodine: A non-randomised, multicentre, open-label, phase 2 trial. The Lancet Oncology. 2016;**17**(9):1272-1282

[38] Shah MH, Wei L, Wirth LJ, Daniels GA, De Souza JA, Timmers CD, et al. Results of randomized phase II trial of dabrafenib versus dabrafenib plus trametinib in BRAF-mutated papillary thyroid carcinoma. Journal of Clinical Oncology. 2017;**35**(15_suppl):6022-6022

[39] Hanna GJ, Busaidy NL, Chau NG, Wirth LJ, Barletta JA, Calles A, et al. Genomic correlates of response to everolimus in aggressive radioiodine-refractory thyroid cancer: A phase II study. Clinical Cancer Research. 2018;**24**(7):1546-1553

[40] Sherman EJ, Ho AL, Fury MG, Baxi SS, Dunn L, Lee JS, et al. Combination of everolimus and sorafenib in the treatment of thyroid cancer: Update on phase II study. Journal of Clinical Oncology. 2015;**33**(15_suppl):6069-6069

[41] Wirth LJ, Sherman E, Robinson B, Solomon B, Kang H, Lorch J,

et al. Efficacy of Selpercatinib in RET-altered thyroid cancers. The New England Journal of Medicine. 2020;**383**(9):825-835

[42] Subbiah V, Hu MIN, Gainor JF, Mansfield AS, Alonso G, Taylor MH, et al. Clinical activity of the RET inhibitor pralsetinib (BLU-667) in patients with RET fusion+ solid tumors. Journal of Clinical Oncology. 2020;**38**(15_suppl):109

[43] Hong DS, DuBois SG, Kummar S, Farago AF, Albert CM, Rohrberg KS, et al. Larotrectinib in patients with TRK fusion-positive solid tumours: A pooled analysis of three phase 1/2 clinical trials. The Lancet Oncology. 2020;**21**(4):531-540

[44] Cabanillas ME, Drilon A, Farago AF, Brose MS, McDermott R, Sohal D, et al. 1916P Larotrectinib treatment of advanced TRK fusion thyroid cancer. Annals of Oncology. 2020;**31**:S1086

[45] Rolfo C, Ruiz R, Giovannetti E, Gil-Bazo I, Russo A, Passiglia F, et al. Entrectinib: A potent new TRK, ROS1, and ALK inhibitor. Expert Opinion on Investigational Drugs. 2015;**24**(11):1493-1500

[46] de Salins V, Loganadane G, Joly C, Abulizi M, Nourieh M, Boussion H, et al. Complete response in anaplastic lymphoma kinase–rearranged oncocytic thyroid cancer: A case report and review of literature. World Journal of Clinical Oncology. 2020;**11**(7):495-503

[47] Grupo Espanol de Tumores Neuroendocrinos. Exploratory Basket Trial of Cabozantinib Plus Atezolizumab in Advanced and Progressive Neoplasms of the Endocrine System. CABATEN Study. clinicaltrials.gov; 2022. Report No.: NCT04400474. Available from: https://clinicaltrials.gov/ct2/show/NCT04400474. [Accessed: May 9, 2022]

[48] Memorial Sloan Kettering Cancer Center. A Pilot Study of the Addition of Cemiplimab, an Antibody to PD-1, to the Treatment of Subjects With BRAF-Mutant Anaplastic Thyroid Cancer Who Are No Longer Responding to Dabrafenib and Trametinib. clinicaltrials.gov; 2021. Report No.: NCT04238624. Available from: https://clinicaltrials.gov/ct2/show/NCT04238624. [Accessed: May 9, 2022]

[49] University of Chicago. Synergy of Pembrolizumab Anti-PD-1 Immunotherapy With Chemotherapy for Poorly Chemo-responsive Thyroid and Salivary Gland Tumors. The iPRIME Study. clinicaltrials.gov; 2022. Report No.: NCT03360890. Available from: https://clinicaltrials.gov/ct2/show/NCT03360890. [Accessed: May 9, 2022]

[50] M.D. Anderson Cancer Center. Lenvatinib in Combination With Pembrolizumab for Stage IVB Locally Advanced and Unresectable or Stage IVC Metastatic Anaplastic Thyroid Cancer. clinicaltrials.gov; 2021. Report No.: NCT04171622. Available from: https://clinicaltrials.gov/ct2/show/NCT04171622. [Accessed: May 9, 2022]

[51] M.D. Anderson Cancer Center. Atezolizumab Combinations With Chemotherapy for Anaplastic and Poorly Differentiated Thyroid Carcinomas. clinicaltrials.gov; 2020. Report No.: NCT03181100. Available from: https://clinicaltrials.gov/ct2/show/NCT03181100. [Accessed: May 9, 2022]

[52] National Cancer Institute (NCI). Phase II Study of XL184 (Cabozantinib) in Combination With Nivolumab and Ipilimumab (CaboNivoIpi) in Patients With Radioiodine-Refractory Differentiated Thyroid Cancer Whose Cancer Progressed After One Prior

VEGFR-Targeted Therapy. clinicaltrials.gov; 2022. Report No.: NCT03914300. Available from: https://clinicaltrials.gov/ct2/show/NCT03914300. [Accessed: May 9, 2022]

[53] Providence Health & Services. Encorafenib/Binimetinib With or Without Nivolumab for Patients With Metastatic BRAF V600 Mutant Thyroid Cancer. clinicaltrials.gov; 2022. Report No.: NCT04061980. Available from: https://clinicaltrials.gov/ct2/show/NCT04061980. [Accessed: May 9, 2022]

[54] M.D. Anderson Cancer Center. Pembrolizumab in Combination With Dabrafenib and Trametinib as a Neoadjuvant Strategy Prior to Surgery in BRAF-Mutated Anaplastic Thyroid Cancer. clinicaltrials.gov; 2021. Report No.: NCT04675710. Available from: https://clinicaltrials.gov/ct2/show/NCT04675710. [Accessed: May 9, 2022]

[55] Academic and Community Cancer Research United. Combination Targeted Therapy With Pembrolizumab and Lenvatinib in Progressive, Radioiodine-Refractory Differentiated Thyroid Cancers: A Phase II Study. clinicaltrials.gov; 2022. Report No.: NCT02973997. Available from: https://clinicaltrials.gov/ct2/show/NCT02973997. [Accessed: May 9, 2022]

[56] Yuliya M. Pembrolizumab in Combination With Standard 1st Line Therapy (Lenvatinib/Chemotherapy) for Locally Advanced or Metastatic Poorly Differentiated or Anaplastic Thyroid Cancer. clinicaltrials.gov; 2021. Report No.: NCT04731740. Available from: https://clinicaltrials.gov/ct2/show/NCT04731740. [Accessed: May 9, 2022]

[57] Sehgal K. A Phase 2 Study of Nivolumab Plus Ipilimumab in RAI Refractory, Aggressive Thyroid Cancer With Exploratory Cohorts in Medullary and Anaplastic Thyroid Cancer. clinicaltrials.gov; 2022. Report No.: NCT03246958. Available from: https://clinicaltrials.gov/ct2/show/NCT03246958. [Accessed: May 9, 2022]

[58] Fudan University. The Efficacy and Safety of Anti-PD-1 Antibody Toripalimab Combined With Surufatinib for Locally Advanced Thyroid Cancer: a Phase II Study. clinicaltrials.gov; 2020. Report No.: NCT04524884. Available from: https://clinicaltrials.gov/ct2/show/NCT04524884. [Accessed: May 9, 2022]

[59] Dongmei J. A Phase II Study to Explore the Safety and Efficacy of Multiple Target Kinase Inhibitor(mTKI) Combined With Anti-Programmed Death-1(PD-1) Antibody in the Treatment of Advanced Thyroid Cancer. clinicaltrials.gov; 2021. Report No.: NCT04521348. Available from: https://clinicaltrials.gov/ct2/show/NCT04521348. [Accessed: May 9, 2022]

[60] Grupo Espanol de Tumores Neuroendocrinos. A Phase II Study of Durvalumab (MEDI4736) Plus Tremelimumab for the Treatment of Patients With Progressive, Refractory Advanced Thyroid Carcinoma—The DUTHY Trial. clinicaltrials.gov; 2022. Report No.: NCT03753919. Available from: https://clinicaltrials.gov/ct2/show/NCT03753919. [Accessed: May 9, 2022]

Chapter 8

Approach and Management of Anaplastic Carcinoma Thyroid

Zuzak Sharafuddin, Rejnish Ravikumar, Malu Rafi, Lekha Madhavan Nair, John Mathew and Kainickal Cessal Thommachan

Abstract

Anaplastic carcinoma thyroid, also known as undifferentiated thyroid carcinoma, is a rare but highly aggressive malignant tumor, which accounts for 2–3% of all thyroid malignancies. It is mostly seen in elderly females in their 6th or 7th decade. It carries a very bad prognosis with an average median survival of 5 months. Patients often present with a rapidly growing, painful, woody hard lower anterior neck mass fixed to underlying structures. In addition to local invasion, patients also present with regional nodal spread and distant metastasis. Though the risk factors for anaplastic carcinoma thyroid are unknown, most of them develop in the setting of long-standing goiter, possibly in an undiagnosed, well-differentiated thyroid carcinoma. Management of anaplastic carcinoma thyroid demands a multidisciplinary approach with the involvement of surgeon, radiation oncologist, radiologist, and endocrinologist. The conventional treatment of anaplastic carcinoma thyroid includes surgery, radiation, and chemotherapy. Recently, multitarget tyrosine kinase inhibitors are also incorporated into the treatment. However, prognosis of the disease is very poor with 4 months of overall survival of 35% and overall disease-specific mortality of 98–99%. In this chapter, we discuss how to approach the condition and various treatment strategies to provide improved treatment outcomes for patients diagnosed with anaplastic carcinoma thyroid.

Keywords: anaplastic carcinoma thyroid, presentation, investigations, surgery, radiation, chemotherapy, targeted agents

1. Introduction

Anaplastic carcinoma thyroid (ATC) is a rare type of thyroid cancer that carries a worse prognosis. It is extremely aggressive, and the average median survival of ATC is 5 months, with less than 20% of the patients alive after 1 year of diagnosis.

2. Epidemiology and pathogenesis

ATC accounts for 1–2% of all thyroid malignancies. It usually affects patients in their 6th to 7th decade with a female predominance (male/female ratio: 1.5:2) [1–3]. However, it contributes up to 14–50% of the annual mortality associated with thyroid cancer [1]. The age-adjusted annual incidence is one to two per million people [4, 5].

Based on different tumor registries, the frequency of ATC is variable in different countries; however, there has been a drastic reduction in its incidence owing to better dietary iodine intake as well as timely diagnosis and treatment of DTC and MNG [1].

ATC usually originates in the background of a long-standing goiter. Dedifferentiation of differentiated thyroid cancer cells is considered the most common cause of ATC. Dedifferentiation arises due to multiple chromosomal aberrations, alteration in signal transduction pathways, and cell-cycle derangement.

BRAF, RAS oncogene, PIK3CA, PTEN, and TP53 mutations are the most commonly associated genetic alterations in ATC [6, 7]. Reduced levels of E-cadherin and beta-catenin are also associated with ATC [8].

Around 20–30% of patients have coexisting differentiated thyroid cancer with papillary being the most common (20%) [9, 10]. Serial biopsies of the thyroid gland also predispose to ATC [11]. Commonly seen mutations and their expression are listed in **Table 1**.

3. Prognosis

ATC carries a dismal prognosis with mortality approaching 100% with 1- and 5-year survival rate less than 30 and 14%, respectively [17–20]. Patients with localized disease have a better prognosis than those with regional or distant metastasis [9, 20]. Tumor size less than 6 cm in maximum dimension carries a better prognosis [9, 18]. Other favorable prognostic factors include unilateral tumor, localized with node-negative or no extrathyroidal extension [16, 20, 21].

Unfavorable factors include older age at diagnosis, male gender, airway compromise during the presentation, and distant metastasis [16, 20].

Mutations associated with ATC (frequency in %) [8]	Expression
TP53 [12]	Upregulated
CTNNB1 [13]	Upregulated
BRAF [14]	Upregulated
RAS [15]	Upregulated
PI3KCA [16]	Downregulated
PTEN [17]	Downregulated
APC [9]	Downregulated

Table 1.
Most common mutations and their expression associated with ATC.

4. Clinical features

The majority of the patients present with a rapidly progressing neck mass with complaints of dysphagia, dyspnea, and neck pain. Approximately 90% will have regional or distant spread at the time of diagnosis [17–19]. The regional spread shows infiltration of perithyroidal fat, lymph nodes, trachea, esophagus, great vessels of the neck, and mediastinum. Based on the infiltration of adjacent neck structures, patients can also develop hoarseness (recurrent laryngeal nerve invasion), Horner's syndrome (parasympathetic chain involvement), and thromboembolic episodes due to carotid infiltration.

Around 40% of patients present with cervical lymphadenopathy and 43% will have distant metastasis most commonly involving lungs followed by bone and brain [20].

Also, patients can present with constitutional symptoms, such as pyrexia of unknown origin, anorexia, weight loss, and rarely with features of thyroiditis [22, 23].

On examination, there will be bilateral but asymmetric enlargement of the thyroid gland with ill-defined borders. Usually, they are nodular, woody hard in consistency, and may be tender. Some nodules may be fluctuant due to focal tumor necrosis [24]. Due to adhesion with the adjacent structures, most of the time the swelling does not move with swallowing. The skin over the swelling may be erythematous and ulcerated.

During clinical examination, they should undergo an ENT evaluation to rule out vocal cord dysfunction or airway compromise.

Other findings include dilated chest wall veins due to superior vena cava obstruction (SVCO) from a retrosternal thyroid growth, stridor due to tracheal invasion, and vocal cord paralysis.

5. Diagnosis

ATC is a very aggressive tumor with a very short doubling time, and hence disease burden should be assessed accurately and promptly.

Laboratory investigations should include a complete blood count, a baseline evaluation of liver and renal function, thyroid function tests, albumin levels, and serum electrolytes levels. Nutritional assessment is also required as most of them will have dysphagia and reduced food intake.

Fine needle aspiration cytology from the thyroid mass can yield an early diagnosis. Morphologic patterns of ATC include spindle cells, pleomorphic giant cells, and squamoid histologies [16]. Most of them will have a mixed morphology of two or all the three patterns and they show extensive necrosis, atypical mitoses, and numerous mitotic figures. However, for immunostaining and molecular studies, a core biopsy is preferred. Routinely they will not stain positive for TTF1, PAX8, and thyroglobulin. Patterns of IHC in various thyroid malignancies are summarized in **Table 2**.

Poorly differentiated carcinoma, large cell lymphoma, and extension of laryngeal carcinoma are the most common differential diagnosis.

Radiological evaluation should be done immediately without any delay. High-resolution ultrasound can be done as it is convenient, rapid, and easy in assessing tumor extent, neck nodes, and adjacent structure involvement.

IHC	DTC	ATC	MTC	SCC	Lymphoma
Pancytokeratin	+++	+++/−	+++	+++	−
Thyroglobulin	+++	−	−	−	−
TTF-1	+++	−/+	+/−	−	−
BRAF v600E	+/-	−/+	−	−	−
PAX8	+++	+/−	+/−	−	−/+
Ki67	<5%	>30%	<20%	>30%	Variable
Chromogranin	−	−	+++	−	−
Calcitonin	−	−	+++/−	−	−
CEA	−	−	+++	−	−
P53	−	+/−	−	+/−	+/−
CD45	−	−	−	−	+++

Table 2.
Patterns of IHC in various thyroid malignancies [25].

Other imaging modalities include CT/MRI of the neck and chest to assess tumor extent and infiltration to adjacent structures. FDG-PET scan has recently gained a role in imaging ATC as it helps in the accurate diagnosis of distant metastasis compared to other imaging modalities [15]. If trachea or esophagus infiltration is suspected, upper GI endoscopy or bronchoscopy is indicated [20, 25].

Molecular testing can be done if available; however, its clinical utility is not well established. Next-generation sequencing should be performed for targetable mutations under the context of a clinical trial. Rapid testing of BRAF V600E mutation is most commonly done if available in FNA or core needle biopsy specimens.

6. Staging

The American Joint Committee on Cancer (AJCC) 8th edition considers all anaplastic cancers as Stage IV. The T category follows the same definitions as those for differentiated thyroid cancers. Intrathyroidal anaplastic cancers form Stage IVA, whereas gross extrathyroidal extension or nodal metastasis form Stage IVB and distant metastasis form Stage IVC.

7. Treatment approach

Initial therapy in these patients mainly depends on the stage of disease and mutation status. Based on this, various treatment options include surgery, radiation with or without chemotherapy, systemic therapy, and palliation.

Gross resection is the main goal in patients with ATC, but the extent of resection should always outweigh the potentially devastating complications and morbidity of the procedures. Airway assessment and prompt treatment without delay are most important. Securing and maintaining a patent airway is challenging in these patients, but, routine tracheostomy is not recommended as it has not shown any improved outcome in survival or quality of life.

Tracheostomy is recommended in impending airway compromise and in those tumors that will not benefit from debulking.

7.1 Stage IVA

Stage IVa includes disease confined within the thyroid capsule. Around 2–15% of patients present with Stage IVa disease, in which, total thyroidectomy with a therapeutic central and lateral neck node dissection is recommended [25, 26]. Attaining gross negative margins have shown a significantly better prognosis than those with tumor residue ($p < 0.005$) [26]. Sugitani et al. reported that, although the benefit from additional therapies for completely resected Stage IVa ATC was not significant, they tend to show better survival with adjuvant radiation compared to those who underwent radical surgery alone (HR: 0.37; 95% CI: 0.121.13; $p = .081$) [27]. However, for completely resected ATC (R0 resection), additional therapies are not routinely indicated.

7.2 Stage IVB

Around 35% of the patients present as Stage IVb with extrathyroidal extension or cervical nodal involvement. They benefit from a combined modality approach.

For resectable tumors, total thyroidectomy with central and lateral therapeutic neck dissection followed by adjuvant chemoradiation has shown significantly prolonged cancer-specific survival compared to those who underwent surgery alone or with adjuvant RT alone (HR: 0.45; 95% CI: 0.250.81; $p = .0083$) [27].

The intensity-modulated RT technique is recommended to get better dose distribution and reduced toxicities [28]. Several authors have reported a dose–response relationship and showed that a dose of more than 60 Gy has shown a good outcome [14, 29, 30]. Commonly delivered radiation dose includes 70 Gy to the gross tumor or 66–70 Gy to the postoperative bed and 54 Gy to the potential microscopic spread region using a standard fractionation schedule [31, 32].

Several chemotherapy agents are used as concurrent, but mostly Doxorubicin 20 mg/m^2 or Paclitaxel 50 mg/m^2 weekly is given [14, 33, 34].

The role of hyperfractionation is not known, as there is poor evidence to show that it is better than conventional fractionation. Also, hyperfractionation is associated with increased toxicity [31, 35, 36].

However, careful patient selection is required as the procedure has an impact on quality of life. Hence, those who get a meaningful clinical benefit should be offered combined modality treatment. The best outcome is seen when adjuvant radiation is started as early as possible, once the patient has recovered from surgery [37].

For unresectable tumors with BRAF mutation, neoadjuvant treatment with Dabrafenib (150 mg twice daily) and Trametinib (20 mg daily) is started to downsize the tumor to facilitate a complete surgical resection [38, 39]. For poor responders of mutation-directed therapies, palliative radiation is an option.

7.3 Stage IVC

Around 55% of ATC patients present with distant metastasis. Stage IVc has no curative treatment and is fatal. One case series has reported a median survival of 4.2 months in those with distant metastasis at presentation compared to 6 months in nonmetastatic ATC [34]. Stage IVc is managed with palliative radiation or debulking with or without systemic therapies.

Palliative resection or debulking should be considered to avoid a future or to treat current airway compromise, which may prolong and improve quality of life. As discussed initially, most of the patients are in their 6th or 7th decade. Hence, airway preservation is enough for old age life preservation.

Palliative external beam radiotherapy (EBRT) has a definite role in symptom control for those who have unresectable/metastatic diseases. It helps in reducing the growth of neck mass and thereby alleviates the pressure symptoms. Various schedules are there, but commonly followed ones are 20 Gy in 5 fractions or 30 Gy in 10 fractions.

Systemic therapies include cytotoxic agents, targeted agents, and immunotherapies. If patients have another targetable mutation, such as NTRK, RET fusion, or ALK, they should be enrolled in clinical trials in mutation-directed systemic therapy.

8. Role of cytotoxic therapy

Chemotherapy is an important independent prognostic factor associated with improved survival [13, 40, 41]. However, data on comparing different chemotherapy regimens in these patients are very limited and underpowered due to the low incidence and aggressiveness of the tumor. In the absence of molecular abnormalities, most commonly given chemotherapy includes a combination of Paclitaxel and carboplatin, Cisplatin and Doxorubicin, Docetaxel and Doxorubicin, Paclitaxel alone or Doxorubicin alone [25]. The role of the combination of Cisplatin and Doxorubicin as well as Paclitaxel as a single agent is being studied in ATC and has shown moderate response [19]. However, all these are based on fairly small single studies that need further validation.

ATC has a very rapid doubling time of 3–12 days, hence, some authors recommend that the chemotherapy regimens should be administered in shorter intervals, on weekly basis rather giving every 3–4 weeks [3, 31]. Systemic therapy protocols are listed in **Table 3**.

Treatment	Protocols and dose
Chemotherapy [3]	Doxorubicin (20 mg/m^2) + Cisplatin 120 mg/m^2) every 28 days Paclitaxel (175 mg/m^2) + carboplatin AUC 5 every 21 days Paclitaxel 50–100 mg/m^2 + Carboplatin AUC2 weekly Docetaxel 20 mg/m^2 + Doxorubicin 20 mg/m^2 weekly Paclitaxel alone 30–60 mg/m^2 or Docetaxel 20 mg/m^2 weekly
BRAF and MEK inhibitors [42, 43]	Dabrafenib 150 mg twice daily + Trametinib 2 mg once daily
RET inhibitor [44]	Selpercatinib 160 mg twice daily or 120 mg twice daily (if body weight <50 kg)
NTRK inhibitor [45]	Larotrectinib 100 mg twice daily Entrectinib 600 mg once daily
ALK inhibitor [46]	Crizotinib 250 mg twice daily Larotrectinib 100 mg twice daily

Table 3.
Systemic therapy protocols.

9. Role of targeted agents

Primary chemoresistance is a commonly encountered issue in ATC that often results in a bad prognosis. Hence, newer therapeutic agents are being investigated in ATC, targeting various molecular alterations.

As mentioned above, one-fourth of the ATC is associated with mutation of BRAF and RAS [47]. A phase II trial was conducted in BRAF V600E-positive tumors including 36 patients with ATC, where the patients were treated with the BRAF inhibitor Dabrafenib plus the MEK inhibitor Trametinib. The treatment was well tolerated with an ORR of 56% (95% CI, 38.1–72.1%), with three complete responses and a median PFS and OS of 6.7 and 14.5 months, respectively [42, 43]. The combination was FDA approved in 2018 as 1st line therapy for BRAF V600E-positive ATC patients.

Unfortunately, acquired resistance to BRAF inhibitors due to secondary mutation of MAPK pathway or via PI3K/AKT/mTOR pathway is common in ATC, and hence newer targeted agents are needed. Around 2–3% of ATC patients will have a mutation of NTRK, ALK, or RET fusion.

For such mutation-positive ATC, very high response rates are reported with specific inhibitors in various trials. A pooled subgroup analysis of trials investigating the role of Larotrectinib in ATC showed a response rate of 29% in two out of seven patients [45, 48]. Similarly, long-lasting responses were also noted with Selpercatinib and Crizotinib in RET fusion ATC and ALK-rearranged ATC, respectively [44, 46]. However, these are small studies, some are equivalent to case reports and need more validation.

Inhibitors of PI3K/AKT/mTOR pathway like Everolimus were tested but showed no response [49]. Combination of Sorafenib and Temsirolimus also could not demonstrate a durable response [50].

Though anti-angiogenic agents, such as Lenvatinib, are approved in radioiodine refractory thyroid cancers, their role in ATC is controversial. Based on a single-arm phase II study with 51 ATC patients, Lenvatinib showed a median PFS benefit of 7.4 months, a median OS of 10.6 months, and an ORR of 24% [51]. However, a recent prospective phase II Lenvatinib trial was stopped due to futility as the interim analysis reported a very low response rate (2.9%) and survival outcome [52].

10. Role of immunotherapy

ATC shows high expression of PD-1/PDL-1, and hence immunotherapy may be a promising approach in these patients. However, data available on its use in ATC are limited. Many phase II trials are ongoing with immunotherapy alone as well as in combination with other agents.

The combination of Pembrolizumab and Lenvatinib in ATC is evaluated in the phase II trial of ATLEP (Anaplastic Thyroid Carcinoma Lenvatinib Pembrolizumab) study and has shown a partial response of 37.5% [53]. Also, a single institution study by Lorch et al. has reported partial response in one-third of the ATC patients treated with a combination of Ipilimumab and Nivolumab [54].

Another PD-1 inhibitor Spartalizumab was tested by Capdevila et al. in 41 heavily pretreated ATC patients and showed a response rate of 19.6%. The median OS was 5.9 months with 40% alive at 1 year. The median PFS was 1.7 months. The response rate was higher for those who had a greater PDL-1 expression (35%) [55]. But, the drug is not FDA approved and is not commercially available.

Drug	Study design	Number of ATC patients (among total)	Median OS (months)
Sunitinib [12]	Phase II	4/71	NA
Axitinib [56]	Phase II	2/60	NA
Pazopanib [57]	Phase II	15/15	3.7
Imatinib [58]	Phase II	11/11	NA
Gefitinib [59]	Phase II	5/27	NA
Vemurafenib [60]	Phase II	7/122	NA
Fosbretabulin [61]	Phase II	26/26	4.7
Spartalizumab [55]	Phase II	38/42	5.9
Efatutazone + Paclitaxel [62]	Phase 1	15/15	3.3
Fosbretabulin+ carboplatin+ Paclitaxel [63]	Phase II/III	80/80	5.2

Table 4.
Newer drugs and their clinical trials.

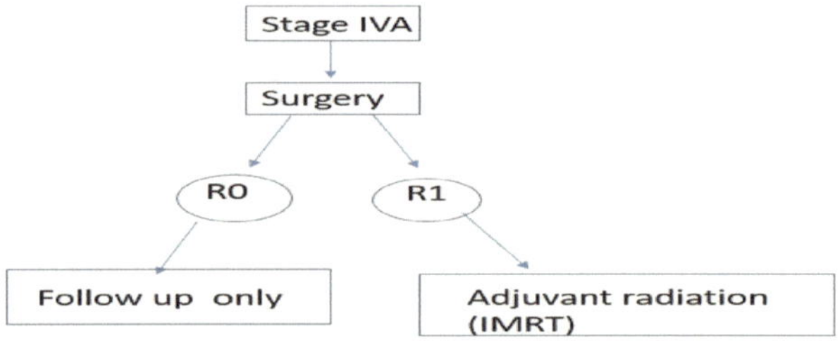

Figure 1.
Stage IVA treatment approach.

Many newer drugs are being tested in phase II and III trials for ATC due to its aggressive nature and poorer outcomes than conventional treatment. A few are listed in **Table 4**.

Stage-wise treatment approach is summarized in **Figures 1–3**. Clinical trials are encouraged and the best supportive care can be considered as an option at any point of treatment.

11. Future directions

Considering the aggressive nature of the disease and its dismal prognosis, novel therapies targeting the signal transduction pathways associated with ATC are to be investigated. Several ongoing trials are being conducted that investigate the role of combining TKIs with immunotherapy or chemotherapy (**Table 5**).

12. End-of-life care

Most of the patients are present in a very advanced stage due to the rapid progression of the disease and will not be eligible for any kind of local or systemic therapy.

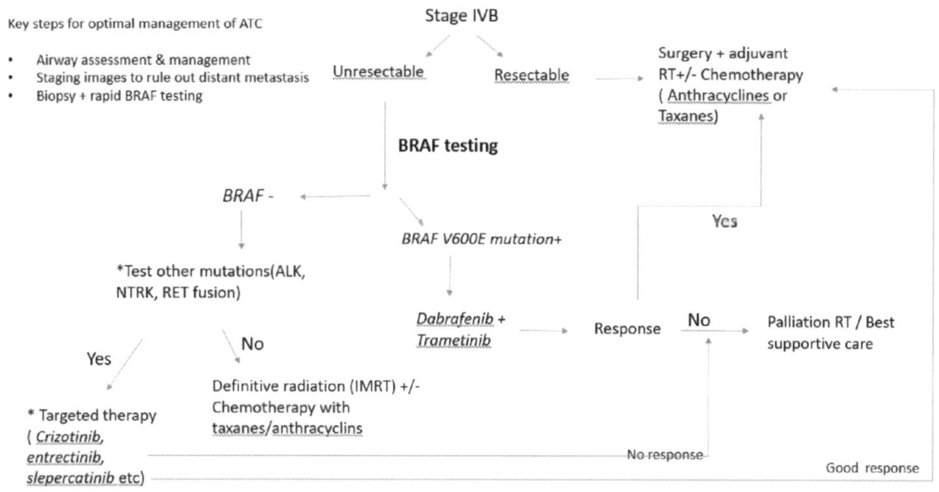

Figure 2.
Stage IVB treatment approach.

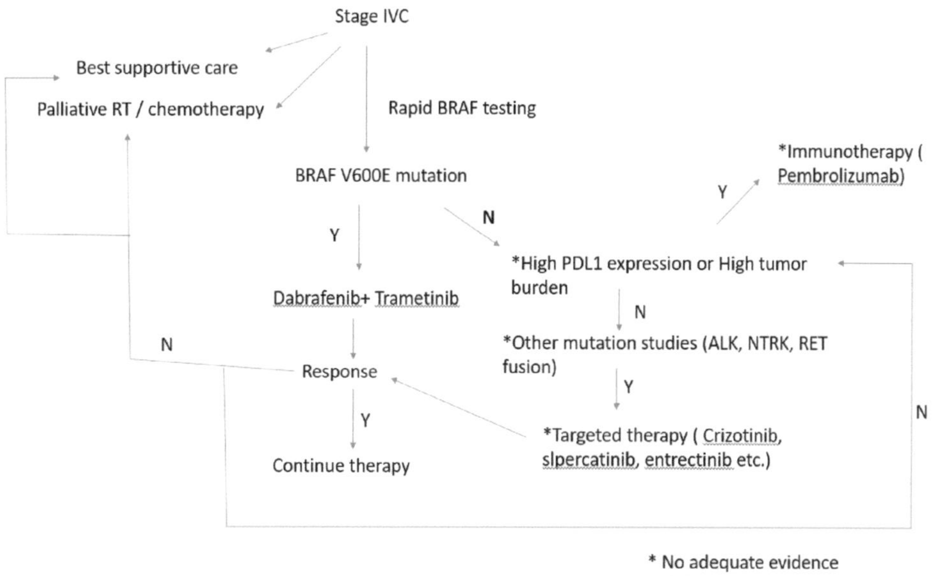

Figure 3.
Stage IV C treatment approach.

End-of-life life care and best supportive care form an integral part of management in these groups of patients [25].

13. Surveillance and follow up

Active surveillance for those who had a complete response to initial treatment is needed. CT of the chest is done within 4 weeks and a single PET–CT is done after 3 months of treatment [15].

Trials	Investigating drug(s)	Phase	Status
NCT03085056 [64]	Trametinib + Paclitaxel in Advanced ATC	Phase 1	Recruiting
NCT02152137 [65]	Efatutazone + Paclitaxel in Advanced ATC	Phase 2	Active, not recruiting
NCT04552769 [66]	Abemaciclib (CDK4/6 inhibitor) in advanced ATC	Phase 2	Recruiting
NCT04675710 [67]	Pembrolizumab + dabrafenib + Trametinib a Neoadjuvant in BRAf mutated ATC	Phase 2	Recruiting
NCT04400474 [68]	Cabozantinib + Atezolizumab in advanced ATC	Phase 2	Recruiting
NCT04579757 [69]	Surufatinib + Tislelizumab in advanced ATC	Phase 1/2	Recruiting
NCT04759911 [70]	Selpercatinib as neoadjuvant in ATC with RET alterations	Phase 2	Recruiting

Table 5.
Ongoing trials in ATC [3].

CT of the neck/chest/abdomen is done thereafter every 1–3 months for the initial 2 years. Later on, less frequent imaging is recommended. Brain imaging is not routinely done, except in case of symptoms of brain metastasis.

There is no role for radioiodine scanning/ablation or serum thyroglobulin measurement.

Thyroid hormone replacement is required for maintaining euthyroid status. T4 should be started (1.6 mcg/kg body weight) immediately after surgery. TSH suppression to less than normal is not indicated in ATC.

14. Conclusion

ATC is a rare thyroid malignancy with an extremely grave prognosis. Diagnosis and treatment should be started quickly and should be based on a multidisciplinary approach, including surgery, radiation, chemotherapy, and targeted agents. Stage IVA tumors should undergo primary surgery with gross-negative margins. For completely resected tumors, there is no role for additional therapies. For resectable stage IVB, surgery followed by adjuvant radiation with or without chemotherapy is recommended. For unresectable tumors, mutation-directed therapies based on BRAF mutation are to be incorporated followed by surgery or radiation. For Stage IVC, palliative treatment is recommended with either palliative radiation or debulking with or without systemic therapies. Although newer mutation-directed therapies are being incorporated into the management of ATC, further validation is needed. The inclusion of novel approaches, such as targeted therapy and immunotherapy either alone or in combination with other modalities, may improve outcomes in these patients.

Author details

Zuzak Sharafuddin, Rejnish Ravikumar, Malu Rafi, Lekha Madhavan Nair, John Mathew and Kainickal Cessal Thommachan*
Department of Radiation Oncology, Regional Cancer Centre, Thiruvananthapuram, Kerala, India

*Address all correspondence to: drcessalthomas@gmail.com

References

[1] Remick SC, Nagaiah G, Hossain A, Mooney CJ, Parmentier J. Anaplastic thyroid cancer: A review of epidemiology, pathogenesis, and treatment. Journal of Oncology. 2011;**2011**:2-5

[2] Siegel RL, Miller KD, Jemal A. Cancer statistics. CA Cancer Journal of Clinical. 2016;**66**(1):7-30

[3] Jannin A, Escande A, al Ghuzlan A, Blanchard P, Hartl D, Chevalier B, et al. Anaplastic thyroid carcinoma: An update. Cancers (Basel). 2022;**14**(4):1-25

[4] Burke JP, Hay ID, Dignan F, Goellner JR, Achenbach SJ, Oberg AL, et al. Long-term trends in thyroid carcinoma: A population-based study in Olmsted County, Minnesota, 1935–1999. Mayo Clinic Proceedings. 2005;**80**(6): 753-758

[5] Davies L, Welch HG. Increasing incidence of thyroid cancer in the United States, 1973–2002. Journal of the American Medical Association. 2006; **295**(18):2164-2167

[6] Pita JM, Figueiredo IF, Moura MM, Leite V, Cavaco BM. Cell cycle deregulation and TP53 and RAS mutations are major events in poorly differentiated and undifferentiated thyroid carcinomas. Journal of Clinical Endocrinology Metabolism. 2014;**99**(3): E497-E507

[7] Charles RP, Silva J, Iezza G, Phillips WA, McMahon M. Activating BRAF and PIK3CA mutations cooperate to promote anaplastic thyroid carcinogenesis. Molecular Cancer Research. 2014;**12**(7):979-986

[8] Smallridge RC, Marlow LA, Copland JA. Anaplastic thyroid cancer: Molecular pathogenesis and emerging therapies. Endocrine-Related Cancer. 2009;**16**(1):17

[9] Nel CJC, van Heerden JA, Goellner JR, Gharib H, McConahey WM, Taylor WF, et al. Anaplastic carcinoma of the thyroid: A clinicopathologic study of 82 cases. Mayo Clinic Proceedings. 1985;**60**(1):51-58

[10] Carcangiu ML, Steeper T, Zampi G, Rosai J. Anaplastic thyroid carcinoma. A study of 70 cases. American Journal of Clinical Pathology. 1985;**83**(2): 135-158

[11] Moore JH, Bacharach B, Choi HY. Anaplastic transformation of metastatic follicular carcinoma of the thyroid. Journal of Surgical Oncology. 1985; **29**(4):216-221

[12] Ravaud A, de la Fouchardière C, Caron P, Doussau A, Do Cao C, Asselineau J, et al. A multicenter phase II study of sunitinib in patients with locally advanced or metastatic differentiated, anaplastic or medullary thyroid carcinomas: Mature data from the THYSU study. European Journal of Cancer. 2017;**76**:110-117

[13] Janz TA, Neskey DM, Nguyen SA, Lentsch EJ. Is the incidence of anaplastic thyroid cancer increasing: A population based epidemiology study. World Journal of Otorhinolaryngology – Head and Neck Surgery. 2019;**5**(1):34-40

[14] Beckham TH, Romesser PB, Groen AH, Sabol C, Shaha AR, Sabra M, et al. Intensity-modulated radiation therapy with or without concurrent chemotherapy in nonanaplastic thyroid cancer with unresectable or gross residual disease. Thyroid. 2018;**28**(9): 1180-1189

[15] Poisson T, Deandreis D, Leboulleux S, Bidault F, Bonniaud G, Baillot S, et al. 18F-fluorodeoxyglucose positron emission tomography and computed tomography in anaplastic thyroid cancer. European Journal of Nuclear Medicine and Molecular Imaging. 2010;**37**(12):2277-2285

[16] Keutgen XM, Sadowski SM, Kebebew E. Management of anaplastic thyroid cancer. Gland Surgery. 2015; **4**(1):44

[17] McIver B, Hay ID, Giuffrida DF, Dvorak CE, Grant CS, Thompson GB, et al. Anaplastic thyroid carcinoma: A 50-year experience at a single institution. Surgery. 2001;**130**(6):1028-1034

[18] Tan RK, Finley RK, Driscoll D, Bakamjian V, Hicks WL, Shedd DP. Anaplastic carcinoma of the thyroid: A 24-year experience. Head & Neck. 1995; **17**(1):41-48

[19] Tennvall J, Lundell G, Wahlberg P, Bergenfelz A, Grimelius L, Åkerman M, et al. Anaplastic thyroid carcinoma: Three protocols combining doxorubicin, hyperfractionated radiotherapy and surgery. British Journal of Cancer. 2002; **86**(12):1848-1853

[20] Kebebew E, Greenspan FS, Clark OH, Woeber KA, McMillan A. Anaplastic thyroid carcinoma: Treatment outcome and prognostic factors. Cancer. 2005;**103**(7):1330-1335

[21] Kihara M, Miyauchi A, Yamauchi A, Yokomise H. Prognostic factors of anaplastic thyroid carcinoma. Surgery Today. 2004;**34**(5):394

[22] Murakami T, Noguchi S, Murakami N, Tajiri J, Ohta Y. Destructive thyrotoxicosis in a patient with anaplastic thyroid cancer. Endocrinologia Japonica. 1989;**36**(6): 905-907

[23] Nishiyama RH, Dunn EL, Thompson NW. Anaplastic spindle-cell and giant-cell tumors of the thyroid gland. Cancer. 1972;**30**(1):113-127

[24] Barr R, Dann F. Anaplastic thyroid carcinoma metastatic to skin. Journal of Cutaneous Pathology. 1974;**1**(5):201-206

[25] Bible KC, Kebebew E, Brierley J, Brito JP, Cabanillas ME, Clark TJ, et al. 2021 American Thyroid Association Guidelines for Management of Patients with Anaplastic Thyroid Cancer. Thyroid. 2021;**31**(3):337-386

[26] Passler C, Scheuba C, Prager G, Kaserer K, Flores JA, Vierhapper H, et al. Anaplastic (undifferentiated) thyroid carcinoma (ATC). A retrospective analysis. Langenbeck's Archives of Surgery. 1999;**384**(3):284-293

[27] Sugitani I, Onoda N, Ito KI, Suzuki S. Management of anaplastic thyroid carcinoma: The Fruits from the ATC Research Consortium of Japan. Journal of Nippon Medical School. 2018;**85**(1): 18-27

[28] Bhatia A, Rao A, Ang KK, Garden AS, Morrison WH, Rosenthal DI, et al. Anaplastic thyroid cancer: Clinical outcomes with conformal radiotherapy. Head & Neck. Jul 2010;**32**(7):829-836

[29] Pezzi TA, Mohamed ASR, Sheu T, Blanchard P, Sandulache VC, Lai SY, et al. Radiation therapy dose is associated with improved survival for unresected anaplastic thyroid carcinoma: Outcomes from the National Cancer Data Base. Cancer. 2017;**123**(9):1653-1661

[30] Mohebati A, Dilorenzo M, Palmer F, Patel SG, Pfister D, Lee N, et al. Anaplastic thyroid carcinoma: A 25-year

single-institution experience. Annals of Surgical Oncology. 2014;**21**(5):1665-1670

[31] De Crevoisier R, Baudin E, Bachelot A, Leboulleux S, Travagli JP, Caillou B, et al. Combined treatment of anaplastic thyroid carcinoma with surgery, chemotherapy, and hyperfractionated accelerated external radiotherapy. International Journal of Radiation Oncology, Biology, Physics. 2004;**60**(4):1137-1143

[32] Kim JH, Leeper RD. Combination adriamycin and radiation therapy for locally advanced carcinoma of the thyroid gland. International Journal of Radiation Oncology, Biology, Physics. 1983;**9**(4):565-567

[33] Baek SK, Lee MC, Hah JH, Ahn SH, Son YI, Rho YS, et al. Role of surgery in the management of anaplastic thyroid carcinoma: Korean nationwide multicenter study of 329 patients with anaplastic thyroid carcinoma, 2000 to 2012. Head & Neck. 2017;**39**(1): 133-139

[34] Ito KI, Hanamura T, Murayama K, Okada T, Watanabe T, Harada M, et al. Multimodality therapeutic outcomes in anaplastic thyroid carcinoma: Improved survival in subgroups of patients with localized primary tumors. Head & Neck. 2012;**34**(2):230-237

[35] Dandekar P, Harmer C, Barbachano Y, Rhys-Evans P, Harrington K, Nutting C, et al. Hyperfractionated Accelerated Radiotherapy (HART) for anaplastic thyroid carcinoma: Toxicity and survival analysis. International Journal of Radiation Oncology, Biology, Physics. 2009;**74**(2):518-521

[36] Wang Y, Tsang R, Asa S, Dickson B, Arenovich T, Brierley J. Clinical outcome of anaplastic thyroid carcinoma treated with radiotherapy of once- and twice-daily fractionation regimens. Cancer. 2006;**107**(8):1786-1792

[37] Smallridge RC, Ain KB, Asa SL, Bible KC, Brierley JD, Burman KD, et al. American Thyroid Association guidelines for management of patients with anaplastic thyroid cancer. Thyroid. 2012;**22**(11):1104-1139

[38] Cabanillas ME, Ferrarotto R, Garden AS, Ahmed S, Busaidy NL, Dadu R, et al. Neoadjuvant BRAF- and immune-directed therapy for anaplastic thyroid carcinoma. Thyroid. 2018;**28**(7): 945-951

[39] Wang JR, Zafereo ME, Dadu R, Ferrarotto R, Busaidy NL, Lu C, et al. Complete surgical resection following neoadjuvant dabrafenib plus trametinib in BRAF V600E-mutated anaplastic thyroid carcinoma. Thyroid. 2019;**29**(8): 1036-1043

[40] Lin B, Ma H, Ma M, Zhang Z, Sun Z, Hsieh IY, et al. The incidence and survival analysis for anaplastic thyroid cancer: A SEER database analysis. American Journal of Translational Research. 2019;**11**(9):5888

[41] Kwon J, Kim BH, Jung HW, Besic N, Sugitani I, Wu HG. The prognostic impacts of postoperative radiotherapy in the patients with resected anaplastic thyroid carcinoma: A systematic review and meta-analysis. European Journal of Cancer. 2016;**59**:34-45

[42] Subbiah V, Cabanillas ME, Kreitman RJ, Wainberg ZA, Cho JY, Keam B, et al. Dabrafenib and trametinib treatment in patients with locally advanced or metastatic BRAF V600-mutant anaplastic thyroid cancer. Journal of Clinical Oncology. 2018;**36**(1): 7-13

[43] Leboulleux S, Lee EK, Bastholt L, Tahara M, Wirth LJ, Sherman SI, et al. Updated efficacy and safety data of dabrafenib (D) and trametinib (T) in patients (pts) with BRAF V600E–mutated anaplastic thyroid cancer (ATC). Annals of Oncology. 2018;**29**: 645-646

[44] Wirth LJ, Sherman E, Robinson B, Solomon B, Kang H, Lorch J, et al. Efficacy of selpercatinib in RET -altered thyroid cancers. The New England Journal of Medicine. 2020;**383**(9): 825-835

[45] Hong DS, DuBois SG, Kummar S, Farago AF, Albert CM, Rohrberg KS, et al. Larotrectinib in patients with TRK fusion-positive solid tumours: A pooled analysis of three phase 1/2 clinical trials. The Lancet Oncology. 2020;**21**(4): 531-540

[46] Godbert Y, De Figueiredo BH, Bonichon F, Chibon F, Hostein I, Pérot G, et al. Remarkable response to crizotinib in woman with anaplastic lymphoma kinase-rearranged anaplastic thyroid carcinoma. Journal of Clinical Oncology. 2015;**33**(20):e84-e87

[47] Cabanillas ME, Zafereo M, Williams MD, Ferrarotto R, Dadu R, Gross N, et al. Recent advances and emerging therapies in anaplastic thyroid carcinoma. F1000Research. 2018;**7**: 511-518

[48] Cabanillas ME, Zafereo M, Gunn GB, Ferrarotto R. Anaplastic thyroid carcinoma: Treatment in the age of molecular targeted therapy. Journal of Oncology Practice/ American Society of Clinical Oncology. 2016;**12**(6):511-518

[49] Lim SM, Chang H, Yoon MJ, Hong YK, Kim H, Chung WY, et al. A multicenter, phase II trial of everolimus in locally advanced or metastatic thyroid cancer of all histologic subtypes. Annals of Oncology. 2013;**24**(12):3089-3094

[50] Sherman EJ, Dunn LA, Ho AL, Baxi SS, Ghossein RA, Fury MG, et al. Phase 2 study evaluating the combination of sorafenib and temsirolimus in the treatment of radioactive iodine-refractory thyroid cancer. Cancer. 2017;**123**(21):4114-4121

[51] Tahara M, Kiyota N, Yamazaki T, Chayahara N, Nakano K, Inagaki L, et al. Lenvatinib for anaplastic thyroid cancer. Frontiers in Oncology. 2017;**7**:3-6

[52] Wirth LJ, Brose MS, Sherman EJ, Licitra L, Schlumberger M, Sherman SI, et al. Open-label, single-arm, multicenter, Phase II trial of lenvatinib for the treatment of patients with anaplastic thyroid cancer. Journal of Clinical Oncology. 2021;**39**(21): 2359-2366

[53] Dierks C, Seufert J, Aumann K, Ruf J, Klein C, Kiefer S, et al. Combination of lenvatinib and pembrolizumab is an effective treatment option for anaplastic and poorly differentiated thyroid carcinoma. Thyroid. 2021;**31**(7):1076-1085

[54] Lorch JH, Barletta JA, Nehs M, Uppaluri R, Alexander EK, Haddad RI, et al. A phase II study of nivolumab (N) plus ipilimumab (I) in radioidine refractory differentiated thyroid cancer (RAIR DTC) with exploratory cohorts in anaplastic (ATC) and medullary thyroid cancer (MTC). Thyroid. 2020;**38**(15): 6513

[55] Wirth LJ, Eigendorff E, Capdevila J, Paz-Ares LG, Lin C-C, Taylor MH, et al. Phase I/II study of spartalizumab (PDR001), an anti-PD1 mAb, in patients with anaplastic thyroid cancer. Cancer. 2018;**36**(15):6024

[56] Zini A, Czerninski R, Sgan-Cohen HD. Oral cancer over four decades: Epidemiology, trends, histology, and survival by anatomical sites. Journal of Oral Pathology & Medicine. 2009;**39**(4): 299-305

[57] Bible KC, Suman VJ, Menefee ME, Smallridge RC, Molina JR, Maples WJ, et al. A multiinstitutional phase 2 trial of pazopanib monotherapy in advanced anaplastic thyroid cancer. The Journal of Clinical Endocrinology and Metabolism. 2012;**97**(9):3179-3184

[58] Ha HT, Lee JS, Urba S, Koenig RJ, Sisson J, Giordano T, et al. A phase II study of imatinib in patients with advanced anaplastic thyroid cancer. Thyroid. 2010;**20**(9):975-980

[59] Pennell NA, Daniels GH, Haddad RI, Ross DS, Evans T, Wirth LJ, et al. A phase II study of gefitinib in patients with advanced thyroid cancer. Thyroid. 2008;**18**(3):317-323

[60] Hyman DM, Puzanov I, Subbiah V, Faris JE, Chau I, Blay J-Y, et al. Vemurafenib in Multiple Nonmelanoma Cancers with BRAF V600 Mutations. The New England Journal of Medicine. 2015;**373**(8):726-736

[61] Mooney CJ, Nagaiah G, Fu P, Wasman JK, Cooney MM, Savvides PS, et al. A phase II trial of fosbretabulin in advanced anaplastic thyroid carcinoma and correlation of baseline serum-soluble intracellular adhesion molecule-1 with outcome. Thyroid. 2009;**19**(3): 233-240

[62] Smallridge RC, Copland JA, Brose MS, Wadsworth JT, Houvras Y, Menefee ME, et al. Efatutazone, an oral PPAR-γ agonist, in combination with paclitaxel in anaplastic thyroid cancer: Results of a multicenter phase 1 trial. The Journal of Clinical Endocrinology and Metabolism. 2013;**98**(6):2392-2400

[63] Sosa JA, Elisei R, Jarzab B, Balkissoon J, Lu SP, Bal C, et al. Randomized safety and efficacy study of fosbretabulin with paclitaxel/carboplatin against anaplastic thyroid carcinoma. Thyroid. 2014;**24**(2):232-240

[64] Sherman E. Trametinib in Combination With Paclitaxel in the Treatment of Anaplastic Thyroid Cancer – Full Text View – ClinicalTrials.gov. MSKCC; 2017. Available from https://clinicaltrials.gov/ct2/show/NCT03085056

[65] Smallridge R. Inolitazone Dihydrochloride and Paclitaxel in Treating Patients With Advanced Anaplastic Thyroid Cancer – Full Text View – ClinicalTrials.gov. Mayo Clinic, National Cancer Institute, Daiichi Sanyo, Inc; 2019. Available from: https://clinicaltrials.gov/ct2/show/NCT02152137

[66] Khanna V. Abemaciclib in Metastatic or Locally Advanced Anaplastic/Undifferentiated Thyroid Cancer – Full Text View – ClinicalTrials.gov. Stanford Cancer Center, University of North Carolina; 2022. Available from: https://clinicaltrials.gov/ct2/show/NCT04552769

[67] Zafereo M. Pembrolizumab, Dabrafenib, and Trametinib Before Surgery for the Treatment of BRAF-Mutated Anaplastic Thyroid Cancer – Full Text View – ClinicalTrials.gov. Anderson Cancer Centre; 2020. Available from: https://clinicaltrials.gov/ct2/show/NCT04675710

[68] Grupo Espanol de Tumores Neuroendocrinos. Trial of Cabozantinib Plus Atezolizumab in Advanced and Progressive Neoplasms of the Endocrine System. The CABATEN Study – Full Text View – ClinicalTrials.gov; 2022.

Available from: https://clinicaltrials.gov/ct2/show/NCT04400474

[69] Kauh J. Surufatinib in Combination With Tislelizumab in Subjects With Advanced Solid Tumors – Full Text View – ClinicalTrials.gov. Hutchison; 2022. Available from: https://clinicaltrials.gov/ct2/show/NCT04579757

[70] Zafereo M. Selpercatinib Before Surgery for the Treatment of RET-Altered Thyroid Cancer – Full Text View – ClinicalTrials.gov. Anderson Cancer Centre; 2021. Available from: https://clinicaltrials.gov/ct2/show/NCT04759911

Chapter 9

Lymph Node Metastasis in Differentiated Thyroid Cancers

Tom Chi-Man Chow and Shirley Yuk-Wah Liu

Abstract

Lymph node metastasis is common in differentiated thyroid cancers. Therapeutic neck dissection removes macroscopic nodal metastasis, reduces local recurrence, and facilitates cancer surveillance. On the other hand, microscopic nodal metastasis is also increasingly recognized as a potential cause of persistent disease or early recurrences. Prophylactic neck dissection, by removing microscopic nodal metastasis, has been proposed to reduce recurrence and prevent future reoperation. When cancer recurs, regional nodal recurrence is most common, and the management should be individualized. We hereby present a narrative review on the management of nodal metastasis in differentiated thyroid cancers.

Keywords: differentiated thyroid cancer, nodal metastasis, neck dissection, therapeutic, prophylactic, recurrent nodal disease

1. Introduction

Differentiated thyroid cancers (DTC) account for over 90% of all thyroid cancers and are further divided into papillary thyroid carcinomas (PTC), follicular thyroid carcinomas (FTC), and Hürthle cell carcinomas. PTC is by far the most common subtype, accounting for 85% of all DTC [1].

1.1 Incidence of lymph node metastasis in DTC

The incidence of lymph node metastasis is different between various types of DTC. PTC is associated with higher frequency of nodal metastasis [2]. On the contrary, FTC seldom metastasizes through the lymphatics [3]. The incidence of nodal metastasis in PTC depends on its detection method and definition. Preoperative imaging can detect nodal disease in up to 30% of patients [4] whereas pathological series reveal nodal metastasis in 20–50% of operated patients [5]. With the replacement of traditional hematoxylin and eosin staining by modern immunohistochemical or molecular genetic techniques, the incidence of nodal micro-metastasis (defined as tumor foci <2 mm) has been reported in up to 90% of patients [6]. Hence nodal metastasis is very common in DTC, particularly amongst patients with PTC and is often underestimated.

1.2 Pattern of lymphatic spread

It is important to understand the pattern of lymphatic spread in DTC as it carries important implications in treatment planning. The prelaryngeal (Delphian) nodes and paratracheal nodes are the most common first sites of nodal metastasis in PTC [7]. Cancer cells then spread laterally to the jugular nodes in a contiguous stepwise fashion prior to spreading to distant sites [8]. If the nodal disease is identified in the lateral neck, both central and lateral neck dissection should be performed. However, "skip metastases", i.e. the presence of lateral nodal disease without central nodal involvement, have been reported in 7–22% of patients with PTC [9, 10]. Multivariate analyses found that skip metastases were most commonly found in patients with unifocal tumor ≤1 cm at the upper one-third of thyroid lobe. Hence, patients without central nodal disease cannot be assumed to be free of lateral nodal metastasis. The knowledge of this pattern of spread enables accurate preoperative assessment of the nodal areas and dictates the necessary extent of neck dissection.

1.3 Classification of cervical lymph nodes

The cervical levels system has been used to accurately communicate the location of nodal disease, standardize terminology in research and guidelines, and define the boundaries of areas where lymph node dissection should be performed. Lymph nodes in the lateral neck compartment are grouped into level I–V, whereas levels VI and VII refer to lymph nodes in the central neck compartment. Several refinements and addition of sublevels were summarized in **Table 1** [11–13].

Nodal level	Anatomical boundaries
IA—submental	Triangular area bounded by the anterior belly of the digastric muscles and hyoid bone
IB—submandibular	Triangular area bounded by the digastric muscle, stylohyoid muscle, and the body of the mandible
IIA/B-upper jugular	Area bounded by stylohyoid muscle anteriorly, the posterior border of the SCM posteriorly, Skull base superiorly, and the hyoid bone inferiorly. The spinal accessory nerve further divides sublevel IIA (anterior) and IIB (posterior)
III—middle jugular	Area bound by hyoid bone superiorly, inferior border of the cricoid cartilage inferiorly, medial border of the SCM anteriorly, and lateral border of the SCM posteriorly.
IV—lower jugular	Area bounded by the inferior border of the cricoid cartilage superiorly, the clavicle inferiorly, medial border of the SCM anteriorly, and lateral border of the SCM posteriorly.
VA/B—posterior triangle	Triangular area bounded by the posterior border of the SCM, trapezius muscle, and the clavicle. The inferior border of the cricoid cartilage further divides sublevel VA (superior) and VB (inferior)
VI—anterior	Area bounded by the hyoid bone superiorly, the suprasternal notch inferiorly, and the anterior border of SCM posteriorly and midline anteriorly.
VII—superior mediastinal	Extension of level VI from suprasternal notch to the level of the innominate artery.

SCM: sternocleidomastoid muscle.

Table 1.
The levels and sublevels of the neck.

1.4 Risk factors predicting nodal metastasis

Understanding the risk factors predicting nodal metastasis in DTC is imperative for identifying the group of patients most vulnerable of nodal metastasis and best indicated for neck dissection. The most consistently reported risk factor for central compartment nodal metastasis is PTC of size larger than 1 cm [14, 15]. The presence of ipsilateral central compartment nodal metastasis is also associated with greater risks of contralateral central compartment involvement. Other reported risk factors include multifocal tumors, extrathyroidal extension, and younger age [14–19]. The only risk factor for lateral compartment nodal metastasis is the presence of central compartment nodal metastasis [19–21].

With advances in molecular techniques, researchers have explored the utility of biomarkers in addition to conventional clinicopathologic features to predict lymph node metastasis in DTC. BRAF is a proto-oncogene which has received frequent attention. Multiple studies have reported the presence of $BRAF^{V600E}$ mutation as a factor associated with nodal metastasis in DTC [22–24]. Yet, other studies have refuted such associations [25, 26]. To date, only seven heterogenous prospective studies have been published but with conflicting conclusions [27–33]. Hence, the true utility of $BRAF^{V600E}$ mutation in risk stratifying nodal metastasis in clinically node negative (cN0) patients remains controversial.

Another potential prognostic marker of differentiated thyroid cancer is the Telomerase Reverse Transcription (TERT) promoter gene which regulates chromosomal integrity. The somatic mutation TERT-C228T was found in up to 11% of DTC [34]. PTC with TERT-C228T was associated with more aggressive tumor behaviors and poorer clinical outcomes when compared with patients exhibiting BRAF mutation alone [35]. The presence of TERT-C228T mutation has been found to be associated with nodal metastasis with an OR of 1.5–1.8 but its prospective role in stratifying patients for neck dissection remains to be elucidated [36, 37].

1.5 Detection of lymph node metastasis in DTC

1.5.1 Incidence of nonpalpable nodal metastasis

Targeted physical examination of the neck is the important first step in detecting nodal metastasis in DTC but its sensitivity is variable. Palpable nodal disease has been reported in only around 5–10% of patients but the incidence of nonpalpable nodal metastasis is much higher. Mayo Clinic reported that ultrasonography (USG) detected nonpalpable nodal metastasis in up to 32% of their PTC cohort [4]. Particularly amongst patients with prior neck surgery, the nonpalpable nodal disease was up to 28 and 64% for the central and lateral compartment, respectively. This highlights the importance of preoperative radiological assessment for nodal metastasis.

1.5.2 Role of USG and computer tomography in the detection of nodal metastasis

USG and computed tomography (CT) are commonly used for preoperative detection of nodal metastasis in DTC. However, it is important to determine which individual imaging modality should be chosen alone or in combination. In general, USG is cheap, easily accessible, and allows diagnostic real-time fine needle aspiration cytology or biopsy. Conversely, CT is a standardized technique that is non-operator-dependent, provides greater anatomical details, and allows accurate evaluation of the retropharyngeal, retrosternal, and mediastinal areas not accessible by USG [38]. In addition, CT can be useful in evaluating extra-thyroidal tumor extension, better detecting multi-level nodal involvement or presence of extranodal extension, and better assessing the anatomical relationship with adjacent critical structures. Hence, both USG and CT are complementary modalities for the investigation of nodal metastasis.

In a retrospective study, USG had an overall sensitivity of 51% and specificity of 92% in preoperative detection of nodal metastasis [39]. The performance of CT was statistically similar at a sensitivity of 62% and a specificity of 93%. Combined USG/CT only improved sensitivity in patients with lateral compartment nodal disease and in patients with nodal involvement of more than one level. These findings were replicated and summarized in a meta-analysis of 1691 patients [40].

Based on the above evidence, the American Thyroid Association (ATA) recommends USG as the first line modality in all DTC while additional CT is considered in larger cancers for patients with higher chance of nodal metastasis and extrathyroidal spread [41]. Scenarios, where CT would be particularly useful, include patients presenting with pressure symptoms arising from thyroid mass, hoarseness of voice, clinically fixative thyroid mass (cT4), and retrosternal thyroid extension incompletely assessed by USG, and patients with palpable bulky lymph nodes.

1.5.3 Role of positron emission tomography in the evaluation of nodal metastasis

Recently there is an increasing interest in the role of positron emission tomography (PET) with 18-fluoro-2-deoxy-d-glucose (^{18}FDG) for evaluating nodal metastasis in DTC. In the last two decades, ^{18}FDG-PET has emerged as a growing method for detecting DTC recurrences, particularly in non-iodine avid diseases such as Hürthle cell carcinomas [42, 43]. In a multicentre study, the sensitivity of ^{18}FDG-PET to detect recurrent disease was shown to be greater than ^{131}I whole body scan (WBS) [44]. However, PET provides low spatial resolution and suboptimal anatomical details. Co-registering PET with CT overcomes this limitation such that ^{18}FDG -PET/CT has become an adjunctive tool in the detection of recurrent DTC, particularly in patients with elevated serum thyroglobulin and negative WBS.

The potential role of PET/CT in the detection of nodal metastasis prior to initial surgery has growing research attention. Jeong et al. evaluated the utility of preoperative PET/CT in their retrospective cohort and reported that PET/CT had a diagnostic accuracy of 92.3% with a sensitivity of 30% and a specificity of 96% in detecting nodal metastasis which was comparable to USG and CT [45]. However, PET/CT did not provide any superior diagnostic accuracy when indirectly compared with USG and CT in a network meta-analysis [46]. Further high-quality direct comparative studies are required to further elucidate the role of PET/CT particularly in the preoperative assessment for nodal metastasis. Current evidence only supports the role of PET/CT in the postoperative detection of recurrent DTC.

Table 2 summarizes the diagnostic performance of various radiological modalities in the preoperative detection of cervical nodal metastasis across all cervical levels.

1.6 Prognostic implication of nodal metastasis

It is important to understand how nodal metastasis in DTC affect prognosis in order to justify its preoperative detection and neck dissection. Although survival

Level I–VI	Sensitivity (%)	Specificity (%)	PPV (%)	NPV (%)	Accuracy (%)
USG	51	92	81	76	77
CECT	62	93	84	80	81
USG + CECT	66	88	77	81	79
^{18}FDG-PETCT	30	96	61	89	87

PPV: positive predictive value; NPV: negative predictive value; and CECT: contrast enhanced CT.

Table 2.
Imaging modalities in preoperative detection of cervical nodal metastasis.

of DTC is generally very good, certain specific populations may suffer from greater chances of recurrence and mortality.

1.6.1 Lymph node metastasis and cancer-specific survival

Regional nodal metastasis had been implicated as a prognostic factor for survival in earlier studies involving large retrospective cohorts [47–49]. For example, Podnos et al. demonstrated a significantly lower overall survival at 14 years (79% vs. 82%) for node-positive patients in their cohort of 9904 patients. However, these studies have been challenged by newer reports that nodal metastasis only adversely affected cancer-specific survival in a subset of patients >45 years of age but not in those <45 years [50].

1.6.2 Lymph node metastasis and disease recurrence

Regional nodal metastasis also had been implicated as a predictor of disease recurrence. Macroscopic lymph node involvement, i.e. clinically palpable or radiologically detectible metastatic lymph node, is associated with a high rate of local recurrence (10–42 percent) [51]. Furthermore, patients with >5 positive lymph nodes, higher lymph node ratio, and the presence of extranodal extension were associated with even higher risks of local disease recurrence [51, 52]. However, the association of microscopic (radiologically undetectable and nonpalpable) nodal disease and recurrence was not well demonstrated [53–56]. A randomized controlled trial of clinically node negative (cN0) patients showed that microscopic nodal disease detected by prophylactic neck dissection did not affect disease-free survival [57].

1.6.3 Lymph node metastasis in staging systems

Based on how nodal metastasis affects survival and recurrence, the presence of nodal metastasis upstages patients over the age of 45 years from American Joint Committee on Cancers (AJCC 6th and 7th edition) from stage I to stage III disease [58]. Similarly, the proposed modifications of the American Thyroid Association risk stratification system classified <5 microscopic nodal metastasis as a component of low-risk disease, macroscopic nodal metastasis or >5 microscopic nodal metastasis as intermediate-risk disease, and any nodal metastasis > = 3 cm in greatest dimension as high-risk disease [59]. These staging systems influence the degree of postoperative thyroid-stimulating hormone suppression therapy and determine whether radioiodine ablation (RAI) should be given. Hence, accurate nodal status has an important clinical significance.

2. Management of lymph node metastasis in initial surgery for DTC

2.1 Classification and types of neck dissection

The management of nodal metastasis must be discussed with clear definitions of various types of lymph node involvement:

i. Clinically node positive/negative (cN+/0) denotes patients with/without clinically or radiologically detected preoperative lymph node involvement

ii. Pathological node positive/negative (pN+/0) denotes patients with/without histoanatomical findings of malignant cell foci (>2 mm in macrometastasis, 200 μm–2 mm in micrometastasis, <2 μm in isolated tumor cells)

iii. Occult nodal metastasis (cN0-pN+) denotes patients with nonpalpable radiologically non-detectable nodal involvement. This is synonymously referred to as microscopic metastasis in literature.

In cN+ patients, lymphadenectomy is referred to as therapeutic neck dissection. Whereas in cN0 patients, lymphadenectomy is referred to as prophylactic neck dissection. The distinction between prophylactic and therapeutic neck dissection cannot be overemphasized as the impact of clinically detectible macroscopic nodal involvement is different from microscopic metastasis in cN0-pN+ disease.

Neck dissection is also classified by the lymphadenectomy extent (**Table 3**) [13]. Selective neck dissection is increasingly performed as the growing knowledge of the pattern of spread of various cancers enables surgeons to spare the lymph node levels not considered at risk of nodal metastasis. Selective neck dissection has been traditionally further classified into supraomohyoid neck dissection (level I–III), central neck dissection (level VI), lateral neck dissection (level II–IV), and posterolateral neck dissection (level II–V). However, these selective neck dissection terminologies were confusing and obsolete with variable inclusion or exclusion of certain levels and sublevels. Hence, selective neck dissection is better described by specifying the levels and sublevels included [13].

Radical neck dissection	The basic standard procedure for cervical lymphadenectomy. All other types of neck dissection are alterations of this procedure. Level I–V lymph nodes are removed together with the IJV, SAN, and the SCM.
Modified radical neck dissection	Preservation of one or more non-lymphatic structure including the IJV, SAN, SCM, or the combination.
Selective neck dissection	Preservation of all of IJV, SAN, and SCM and one or more lymph node levels based on the pattern of spread of the malignancy.

IJV: internal jugular vein; SAN: spinal accessory nerve; and SCM: sternocleidomastoid muscle.

Table 3.
Classification of neck dissections.

2.2 Therapeutic neck dissection

Therapeutic neck dissection is performed when patients have preoperatively confirmed nodal metastasis (cN+). It can be performed during initial thyroidectomy or as a staged secondary procedure after initial thyroidectomy.

2.2.1 When nodal metastasis was detected in the central compartment preoperatively

For DTC with preoperatively confirmed central compartment nodal metastasis, therapeutic central neck dissection should be performed bilaterally. This should extend superiorly from the hyoid bone to the innominate artery inferiorly. It is laterally bound by bilateral carotid arteries, anteriorly bound by the superficial layer of the deep cervical fascia, and posteriorly bound by the deep layer of the deep cervical fascia [12]. A compartment-oriented lymphadenectomy with the removal of all fibroadipose tissues within the compartment while identifying and preserving the ipsilateral recurrent laryngeal nerve (RLN), superior, and inferior parathyroid glands should be performed. In the past, non-anatomical nodal dissection ("berry picking") was performed but studies have shown a significantly greater recurrences rate (100% vs. 9%) with non-anatomical dissection versus compartment-oriented dissection, and similar surgical morbidities [60].

The most common morbidities of central neck dissection are transient hypocalcaemia (4–60%) and transient RLN injury (0–5%) but permanent hypocalcaemia and permanent RLN injury can occur in up to 15 and 12% of patients, respectively [61]. Although isolated studies demonstrated no additional complication risk from extra central neck dissection, most series had reported higher rates of complication when central neck dissection was performed concurrently with thyroidectomy and the outcomes were associated with surgeon's experience [62–65].

2.2.2 When nodal metastasis was detected in the lateral compartment preoperatively

For DTC with preoperatively confirmed lateral compartment nodal disease, the chance of concomitant central compartment disease is high. Therefore, patients should undergo both therapeutic lateral and concomitant central neck dissection.

The extent of therapeutic lateral neck dissection is not well agreed upon. While the consensus statement from the ATA recommends the removal of levels IIA, III, IV, and VB in a comprehensive therapeutic neck dissection, other authors routinely recommend a full dissection of levels II–V [11]. In DTC, the rate of nodal metastasis at the various lateral neck levels differs widely. The incidence of nodal metastasis at level III (62–67%) and level IV (50–67%) were significantly higher than that at level II (42–56%) and level V (29–40%) [21, 66–68]. A further distinction of sublevels IIA/B and VA/B were reported. Farrag et al. stated that level IIB rarely had nodal metastasis (8.5%) while all level V metastases were within level VB [68]. Others reported that level IIB nodal metastasis was exclusively accompanied by level IIA nodal metastasis [68, 69]. To date, no randomized controlled trials were published to determine the most appropriate operative extent. But available evidence supports a selective approach where level IIB and VA are only dissected if there is preoperative or intraoperative suspicion of level II or level V involvement. There is an added advantage that avoiding routine level IIB and VA dissection can minimize the risk of spinal accessory nerve injury.

Only a few studies have dealt with the surgical morbidities of lateral neck dissection. Two key complications after lateral neck dissection are lymphatic leakage secondary to thoracic duct damage (0.5–8%), and spinal accessory nerve injury (25–50%) resulting in shoulder dysfunction [27]. Other less common nerve injuries can be related to greater auricular nerve (48%), cervical plexus, sympathetic trunk (5%), and phrenic, hypoglossal, and vagal nerves [28, 63].

2.3 Prophylactic central neck dissection: why and who?

The rationale for prophylactic neck dissection is based on the fact that occult nodal metastasis is common. Despite comprehensive preoperative imaging, there is clinically node-negative (cN0) patients who are found to have unexpected nodal metastasis (pN+) on pathology. The incidence of this occult nodal disease was reported in up to 54% of patients who underwent elective bilateral central neck dissection during total thyroidectomy for DTC [14]. About 50% of which were a bilateral occult nodal disease. Prophylactic neck dissection allows accurate disease staging, improves postoperative risk stratification, and improves serum thyroglobulin levels facilitating postoperative surveillance. Prophylactic neck dissection at the initial thyroid surgery may additionally help to avoid reoperation in the future.

The evidence supporting routine prophylactic central neck dissection is controversial. While some earlier studies reported that prophylactic central neck dissection could reduce the risk of nodal recurrence and cancer-specific survival [29], others did not show such benefit. Aggregating these heterogenous nonrandomized studies, a meta-analysis showed that prophylactic central neck dissection had a lower risk of locoregional recurrence (risk ratio 0.66) than those without neck dissection [30]. However, prophylactic central neck dissection was associated with higher rates of overall morbidity, especially transient hypoparathyroidism. To date, three randomized trials have been published on prophylactic central neck dissection and all failed to show improvement in oncological outcomes or recurrence-free survival [31, 32, 57]. While it was shown that the prevalence of operative morbidities was similar in the group with prophylactic central neck dissection, all these randomized trials were underpowered to demonstrate the difference in survival outcomes and morbidity rates. To this end, ATA examined the feasibility of a multi-institutional prospective randomized controlled trial and concluded that the sample size required would be prohibitively large (>5800) given the low rate of disease recurrence and operative morbidities [33].

Both the ATA guidelines and the American Association of Endocrine Surgeons guidelines recommend a selective approach based on assessment of a patient's risk factors [59, 70]. For patients with T1/2 tumor, the risks of central nodal metastasis are relatively small, and thus prophylactic central neck is not recommended. Patients with T3/4 tumor, or extrathyroidal extension, or BRAF mutation may be considered at higher risk, and option of prophylactic central neck dissection should be considered. The British Thyroid Association on the other hand recommended personalized decision-making for prophylactic central neck dissection on the basis of one or more high-risk factors (adverse histological subtype, age $\geq$ 45 years, multifocal, tumors >4 cm, extra-thyroidal extension). This highlights the variability and uncertainty in this aspect of management of DTC.

2.4 Prophylactic lateral neck dissection

Prophylactic lateral neck dissection is generally not recommended. The rationale is that lateral neck dissection can be deferred until the nodal disease become clinically apparent and proven. The concern to reoperate after initial thyroidectomy is lower as the lateral compartment is not entered during the initial surgery. Evidence suggested that removal of microscopic nodal disease in the lateral department had not been proven to improve cancer-specific or disease-free survival [51]. Considering the morbidity associated with lateral neck dissection, lateral neck dissection is in general reserved for proven nodal disease only.

2.5 Sentinel lymph node biopsy in differentiated thyroid cancer

The concept of sentinel lymph node biopsy (SLNB) depends on the stepwise pattern of lymphatic spread and the belief that the sentinel node (SLN), the first node that drains the tumor, will reflect the status of the remaining lymph nodes within the drainage basin.

2.5.1 Various sentinel lymph node techniques

Various SLNB techniques have been studied in PTC. The use of vital dye was the earliest described technique, but it is growing out of popularity due to its disadvantages that (1) lateral compartment SLN cannot be visualized during thyroidectomy; (2) parathyroid glands may have uptake; and (3) the risks of anaphylaxis [71]. The use of radioisotope as an alternative technique allows identification of SLN located outside the central compartment without parathyroid gland uptake. Furthermore, the addition of SPECT/CT imaging can improve preoperative anatomical localization of the SLN. In a meta-analysis including 45 retrospective studies, the SLN detection rates for vital dye technique, radiolabelled lymphoscintigraphy, vital dye plus lymphoscintigraphy, and lymphoscintigraphy plus SPECT/CT were 83, 96, 87, and 93% respectively, while the reported respective false negative rates were 38, 40, 17, and 8% [72].

2.5.2 Using sentinel lymph node biopsy to guide neck dissection

SLNB has been applied in the management of PTC where SLNB-positive patients can undergo dissection of the involved compartments, and negative patients can be spared the risks and added costs of unnecessary procedure. The negative predictive value of each SLNB technique is the most important parameter to determine whether neck dissection should be performed, and it is dependent on the SLN detection rate and the false negative rate of each technique. Relevant literature data was diversified, firstly due to the difficulty to interpret SLN at frozen section; secondly due to variable definition of the SLN resulting in non-sampling of non-dominant nodes; thirdly due to the occasional skip metastasis; and finally due to the learning curve [73, 74]. Therefore, despite promising initial results from SLNB, further high-quality prospective evidence is necessary. Furthermore, the cost-effectiveness of SLNB strategy also remains ambiguous. A retrospective study reported that the cost of implementing SLNB outweighed the potential cost saving from avoided procedures and morbidities [75]. As such, the current use of SLNB remains within clinical trial settings.

3. Management of recurrent nodal disease

DTC recurs in up to 30% of patients. Three quarters of these recurrences are at the cervical and mediastinal lymph nodes, 20% are in the thyroid remnant and 21% are distant with the lungs being the most common [76]. Although recurrences are common, resultant cancer related deaths are not [77].

3.1 Management of resectable nodal recurrence

When patients develop isolated nodal recurrence after previous surgery, further curative surgery, if technically feasible, confers the advantages of avoiding future local complications arising from the recurrent tumor, improving serum thyroglobulin level, and facilitating RAI treatments.

3.1.1 Low volume recurrences

Although surgical removal of recurrence confers advantages, low volume recurrence does not necessarily require surgery. Several observational studies have suggested that low-volume recurrent nodal disease can be indolent and can be managed with active surveillance. In a retrospective cohort of 166 patients with suspicious lateral compartment lymph node of a median size of 1.3 cm, less than 10% of the patients had interval progression by >5 mm, and 14% had complete resolution [78]. Thyroid stimulating hormone suppression therapy should be continued during active surveillance.

3.1.2 Macroscopic resectable recurrence

Larger volume recurrent nodal disease has been associated with poorer cancer-specific survival and is best treated with revision surgery [79]. In the cases where the recurrence occurs in a previously un-operated neck region, a formal neck dissection should be considered. Revision surgery achieves biochemical remission rates of 21–66%. While most modern series suggest that revision surgery can achieve a high clearance rate of structural disease in over 80% of patients [80].

However, in the cases where recurrence occurs in a previously operated area, the risk of re-operative surgery should be balanced against oncological disease clearance. Re-operative surgery for recurrent nodal disease has higher risk of major complications due to the increased technical demand for dissecting scarred tissue and altered anatomy. The morbidity from re-operative surgery is related to the region undergoing dissection, the experience of surgeons, and the degree of scarring from initial surgery. In general, the incidence of permanent and transient hypoparathyroidism was 0–9.5%, and 0–46.3% respectively. While the rate of transient and permanent unexpected RLN palsy was an average of 3.6 and 1.2%, respectively [81].

3.1.3 Decision-making for re-operative neck dissection

The ATA recommends that radiologically localized, cytology confirmed, recurrent central neck nodes ≥8 mm and lateral neck nodes ≥10 mm in the smallest dimension should be considered for surgery. The exact size threshold for re-operative neck dissection is anecdotal by consensus, and available supporting evidence are scarce. The relationship between the size of recurrent structural disease, morbidity from surgery, and response to therapy had been assessed by Lang et al. in their cohort of 130 patients [82]. Lesion >15 mm was an independent risk factor for incomplete biochemical response. The rates of incomplete surgical resection, unexpected vocal cord palsy, and overall morbidity were also significantly higher in patients with lesions >15 mm than those with lesions <15 mm. Hence, the authors propose that the threshold for continued active surveillance can be less stringent and extended to larger lesions.

Besides the size of recurrence, several other factors are also important to be considered during discussion for revision surgery. These include patient's factors (symptoms arising from recurrent disease, vocal cord status, previous neck irradiation/surgery, motivation for surgery), surgeon's experience, and disease factors (lesion's location in relation to vital structures, factors reflecting tumor aggressiveness such as serum thyroglobulin doubling time, speed of radiological growth, iodine avidity, and the presence of adverse molecular markers) [81]. Hence, such a decision is best discussed with a dedicated multidisciplinary team including surgeons, endocrinologists, nuclear medicine physicians, pathologists, and oncologists [83].

3.2 Nonoperative local treatment for nodal recurrence

Radioactive iodine ablation (RAI) may be employed in patients with ^{131}I-avid low-volume disease detected on WBS or as adjuvant treatment following surgery. To date, no randomized controlled trials had demonstrated superior outcomes with RAI alone or as adjuvant treatment in the setting of locoregional recurrent disease [59]. However, ^{131}I non-avid lesions are unlikely to respond and empirical RAI is not recommended [84].

With a larger volume of nodal recurrences, percutaneous ethanol injection (PEI) for metastatic cervical lymph node was first reported in the early 1990s–2000s [85]. Studies have reported sonographic successful ablation in up to 84% of treated lymph nodes after repeated sessions of treatment [86]. Most ablated lymph nodes decreased in size and 46% completely disappeared [87]. Radiofrequency ablation (RFA) for metastatic cervical lymph node is another newer modality of nonoperative treatment for recurrent nodal disease. It has been associated with a greater mean volume reduction of 55–95% and complete resolution of the structural lesion in 40–60% [88]. The limitation of these ablative modalities is that only limited small studies are available. They are considered a nonoperative form of lymph node picking and, as such, are best considered in patients with high surgical risks or those who declined surgery.

3.3 Management of extensive/unresectable nodal recurrence

Advanced nodal recurrence may involve extensive soft-tissues with potential laryngeal, tracheal, esophageal, or carotid sheath invasion. While there is no strict description to define unresectable diseases, extensive organ resections such as hemi- or total laryngectomies, circumferential tracheal resection, and esophagectomies have been described [89]. The related morbidity and the anticipated functional impairment must be accepted by the patient. Even in patients with distant metastases and concomitant loco-regional recurrent disease compromising the aerodigestive tract, palliative re-operative surgery may be considered on a case-by-case basis, followed by adjuvant RAI treatment [90].

In extensive unresectable nodal recurrences, RAI alone is unlikely able to eradicate the disease as the absorbed radiation dose is generally inadequate. External beam radiotherapy (EBRT) can be considered for locoregional control in such patients. However, acute treatment-related morbidities, including dermatitis, mucositis, and dysphagia, are not uncommon and efficacy has only been reported in retrospective cohorts [91]. To date, there are no randomized trials that address specific indications for EBRT in patients with recurrent DTC. Hence, individual practice is variable.

3.3.1 Other systemic treatment for extensive/unresectable recurrent diseases

Patients with gross symptomatic recurrent disease that cannot be alleviated with surgery or EBRT or had become RAI refractory, are candidates for systemic therapy. Inhibition of protein kinases that function in key signaling pathways can regulate tumor proliferation, angiogenesis, metastasis, and apoptosis. Furthermore, inhibition of kinases involved in the mitogen-activated protein kinase pathway has been shown to re-express genes of iodine metabolism and thus allow restoration of RAI uptake in RAI refractory DTC [92]. Somatic mutation testing can be performed to identify oncogenic targets such as gene rearrangements in NTRK, RET, or BRAF. This may guide the use of mutation-specific kinase inhibitor such as TRK inhibitors (e.g. Larotrectinib, Entrectinib) and RET inhibitors (e.g. Selpercatinib, Pralsetinib). However, BRAF inhibitors (e.g. Vemurafenib, Dabrafenib) are currently nonapproved in thyroid cancers and have been used off-labeled.

Given the high cost of performing mutation analysis and the limited participation in clinical trials, anti-angiogenic multi-kinase inhibitors (aaMKI) such as Lenvatinib or Sorafenib are alternative agents. No head-to-head comparisons of aaMKI are available. Most of these aaMKI target vascular endothelial growth factor receptors (VEGFR) in angiogenic pathways. Of note, patients with risks of bleeding e.g. recent major surgery, haemorrhagic brain metastasis, or recent thromboembolic events are relatively contraindicated for MKI. Furthermore, tracheoesophageal fistulation have been reported in patients with prior EBRT and MKI treatment.

If a patient is intolerant to, or the disease is refractory to kinase inhibitors, conventional cytotoxic agents (e.g. Doxorubicin) may be alternative options but experience is sparse.

4. Conclusions

Nodal metastasis is common in differentiated thyroid cancers and its pattern of spread is well recognized. Despite improvements in technology, imaging has limited sensitivity to detect nodal metastasis before initial surgery or when disease recurs. Occult nodal metastasis is very common and may explain persistent disease or early recurrence. However, distinction between macroscopic and microscopic nodal metastasis and their prognostic implications must be made clear.

Many unanswered questions regarding management of nodal metastasis remain. Prophylactic central neck dissection may remove occult nodal metastasis but its impact on survival lacks high-quality evidence support and is best reserved for selected patients by experts. Sentinel nodal biopsy is an attractive concept but further evidence from research is required. Even when nodal metastasis is detected before the initial surgery, the optimal extent of therapeutic neck dissection remains debated. When disease ultimately recurs, the decision to operate is complex, taking into consideration the increased rate of morbidities in re-operative surgeries. Active surveillance may be best for low-volume recurrent disease while other nonoperative treatments can be considered in patients not suitable for surgery.

Conflict of interest

The authors declare no conflict of interest.

Author details

Tom Chi-Man Chow and Shirley Yuk-Wah Liu*
Division of Endocrine Surgery, Department of Surgery, Prince of Wales Hospital, Chinese University of Hong Kong, Hong Kong SAR, China

*Address all correspondence to: liuyw@surgery.cuhk.edu.hk

References

[1] Hundahl SA, Fleming ID, Fremgen AM, Menck HR. A national cancer data base report on 53,856 cases of thyroid carcinoma treated in the U.S., 1985-1995. Cancer. 1998;**83**(12):2638-2648

[2] Lang W, Borrusch H, Bauer L. Occult carcinomas of the thyroid. Evaluation of 1020 sequential autopsies. American Journal of Clinical Pathology. 1988;**90**(1):72-76

[3] Zaydfudim V, Feurer ID, Griffin MR, Phay JE. The impact of lymph node involvement on survival in patients with papillary and follicular thyroid carcinoma. Surgery. 2008;**144**(6):1070-1078

[4] Stulak JM, Grant CS, Farley DR, Thompson GB, Van Heerden JA, Hay ID, et al. Value of preoperative ultrasonography in the surgical management of initial and reoperative papillary thyroid cancer. Archives of Surgery. 2006;**141**(5):489-496

[5] Grebe SK, Hay ID. Thyroid cancer nodal metastases: Biologic significance and therapeutic considerations. Surgical Oncology Clinics of North America. 1996;**5**(1):43-63

[6] Qubain SW, Nakano S, Baba M, Takao S, Aikou T. Distribution of lymph node micrometastasis in pN0 well-differentiated thyroid carcinoma. Surgery. 2002;**131**(3):249-256

[7] Noguchi S, Noguchi A, Murakami N. Papillary carcinoma of the thyroidI. Developing pattern of metastasis. Cancer. 1970;**26**(5):1053-1060

[8] Kim H, Kim TH, Choe JH, Kim JH, Kim JS, Oh YL, et al. Patterns of initial recurrence in completely resected papillary thyroid carcinoma. Thyroid. 2017;**27**(7):908-914

[9] Park JH, Lee YS, Kim BW, Chang HS, Park CS. Skip lateral neck node metastases in papillary thyroid carcinoma. World Journal of Surgery. 2012;**36**(4):743-747

[10] Ryu YJ, Kwon SY, Lim SY, Na YM, Park MH. Predictive factors for skip lymph node metastasis and their implication on recurrence in papillary thyroid carcinoma. Biomedicine. 2022;**10**(1):179

[11] Stack BC, Ferris RL, Goldenberg D, Haymart M, Shaha A, Sheth S, et al. American thyroid association consensus review and statement regarding the anatomy, terminology, and rationale for lateral neck dissection in differentiated thyroid cancer. 2022. Available from: www.liebertpub.com

[12] Carty SE, Cooper DS, Doherty GM, Duh QY, Kloos RT, Mandel SJ, et al. Consensus statement on the terminology and classification of central neck dissection for thyroid cancer. 2022. Available from: www.liebertpub.com

[13] Thomas Robbins K, Clayman G, Levine PA, Medina J, Sessions R, Shaha A, et al. Neck dissection classification update: Revisions proposed by the American head and neck society and the american academy of otolaryngology-head and neck surgery. Archives of Otorhinolaryngology-Head & Neck Surgery. 2002;**128**(7):751-758

[14] Koo BS, Choi EC, Yoon YH, Kim DH, Kim EH, Lim YC. Predictive factors for ipsilateral or contralateral central lymph node metastasis in unilateral papillary

thyroid carcinoma. Annals of Surgery. 2009;**249**(5):840-844

[15] Roh JL, Kim JM, Park CI. Central lymph node metastasis of unilateral papillary thyroid carcinoma: Patterns and factors predictive of nodal metastasis, morbidity, and recurrence. Annals of Surgical Oncology. 2011;**18**(8):2245-2250

[16] Yip L, Nikiforova MN, Carty SE, Yim JH, Stang MT, Tublin MJ, et al. Optimizing surgical treatment of papillary thyroid carcinoma associated with BRAF mutation. Surgery. 2009;**146**(6):1215-1223

[17] Yang JR, Song Y, Chang SJ, Shi LL. Prediction of central compartment nodal metastases in papillary thyroid cancer using TI-RADS score, blood flow, and multifocality. Acta Radiologica: Diagnosis (Stockh). 2021:2841851211041811. DOI: 10.1177/02841851211041811 [published online ahead of print, 2021 Nov 29]

[18] Joo JY, Park JY, Yoon YH, Choi B, Kim JM, Jo YS, et al. Prediction of occult central lymph node metastasis in papillary thyroid carcinoma by preoperative BRAF analysis using fine-needle aspiration biopsy: A prospective study. The Journal of Clinical Endocrinology and Metabolism. 2012;**97**(11):3996-4003

[19] Feng JW, Yang XH, Wu BQ, Sun DL, Jiang Y, Qu Z. Predictive factors for central lymph node and lateral cervical lymph node metastases in papillary thyroid carcinoma. Clinical and Translational Oncology. 2019;**21**(11):1482-1491

[20] Zhang L, Wei WJ, Ji QH, Zhu YX, Wang ZY, Wang Y, et al. Risk factors for neck nodal metastasis in papillary thyroid microcarcinoma: A study of 1066 patients. The Journal of Clinical Endocrinology and Metabolism. 2012;**97**(4):1250-1257

[21] Liu C, Xiao C, Chen J, Li X, Feng Z, Gao Q, et al. Risk factor analysis for predicting cervical lymph node metastasis in papillary thyroid carcinoma: A study of 966 patients. BMC Cancer. 2019;**19**(1):622

[22] Howell GM, Nikiforova MN, Carty SE, Armstrong MJ, Hodak SP, Stang MT, et al. BRAF V600E mutation independently predicts central compartment lymph node metastasis in patients with papillary thyroid cancer. Annals of Surgical Oncology. 2013;**20**(1):47-52

[23] Xing M, Alzahrani AS, Carson KA, Viola D, Elisei R, Bendlova B, et al. Association between BRAF V600E mutation and mortality in patients with papillary thyroid cancer. Journal of the American Medical Association. 2013;**309**(14):1493-1501

[24] Kim TH, Park YJ, Lim JA, Ahn HY, Lee EK, Lee YJ, et al. The association of the BRAF(V600E) mutation with prognostic factors and poor clinical outcome in papillary thyroid cancer: A meta-analysis. Cancer. 2012;**118**(7):1764-1773

[25] Gouveia C, Can NT, Bostrom A, Grenert JP, van Zante A, Orloff LA. Lack of association of BRAF mutation with negative prognostic indicators in papillary thyroid carcinoma: The University of California, San Francisco, experience. JAMA Otolaryngology–Head & Neck Surgery. 2013;**139**(11):1164-1170

[26] Lee KC, Li C, Schneider EB, Wang Y, Somervell H, Krafft M, et al. Is BRAF mutation associated with lymph node metastasis in patients with papillary thyroid cancer? Surgery. 2012;**152**(6):977-983

[27] Dralle H, Machens A. Surgical management of the lateral neck

compartment for metastatic thyroid cancer. Current Opinion in Oncology. 2013;**25**(1):20-26

[28] Welch K, McHenry CR. Selective lateral compartment neck dissection for thyroid cancer. The Journal of Surgical Research. 2013;**184**(1):193-199

[29] Barczyński M, Konturek A, Stopa M, Nowak W. Prophylactic central neck dissection for papillary thyroid cancer. The British Journal of Surgery. 2013;**100**(3):410-418

[30] Zhao W, You L, Hou X, Chen S, Ren X, Chen G, et al. The effect of prophylactic central neck dissection on locoregional recurrence in papillary thyroid cancer after total thyroidectomy: A systematic review and meta-analysis: pCND for the locoregional recurrence of papillary thyroid cancer. Annals of Surgical Oncology. 2017;**24**(8):2189-2198

[31] Sippel RS, Robbins SE, Poehls JL, Pitt SC, Chen H, Leverson G, et al. A randomized controlled clinical trial: No clear benefit to prophylactic central neck dissection in patients with clinically node negative papillary thyroid cancer. Annals of Surgery. 2020;**272**(3):496-503

[32] Ahn JH, Kwak JH, Yoon SG, Yi JW, Yu HW, Kwon H, et al. A prospective randomized controlled trial to assess the efficacy and safety of prophylactic central compartment lymph node dissection in papillary thyroid carcinoma. Surgery. 2022;**171**(1):182-189

[33] Carling T, Carty SE, Ciarleglio MM, Cooper DS, Doherty GM, Kim LT, et al. American Thyroid Association design and feasibility of a prospective randomized controlled trial of prophylactic central lymph node dissection for papillary thyroid carcinoma. American Thyroid Association. 2012;**22**(3):237-244

[34] Liu X, Bishop J, Shan Y, Pai S, Liu D, Murugan AK, et al. Highly prevalent TERT promoter mutations in aggressive thyroid cancers. Endocrine-Related Cancer. 2013;**20**(4):603-610

[35] Liu R, Li Y, Chen W, Cong J, Zhang Z, Ma L, et al. Mutations of the TERT promoter are associated with aggressiveness and recurrence/ distant metastasis of papillary thyroid carcinoma. Oncology Letters. 2020;**20**(4):1

[36] Yang J, Gong Y, Yan S, Chen H, Qin S, Gong R. Association between TERT promoter mutations and clinical behaviors in differentiated thyroid carcinoma: A systematic review and meta-analysis. Endocrine. 2020;**67**(1):44-57

[37] Liu C, Liu Z, Chen T, Zeng W, Guo Y, Huang T. TERT promoter mutation and its association with clinicopathological features and prognosis of papillary thyroid cancer: A meta-analysis. Scientific Reports. 2016;**6**(1):36990

[38] Lesnik D, Cunnane ME, Zurakowski D, Acar GO, Ecevit C, MacE A, et al. Papillary thyroid carcinoma nodal surgery directed by a preoperative radiographic map utilizing CT scan and ultrasound in all primary and reoperative patients. Head & Neck. 2014;**36**(2):191-202

[39] Kim E, Park JS, Son KR, Kim JH, Jeon SJ, Na DG. Preoperative diagnosis of cervical metastatic lymph nodes in papillary thyroid carcinoma: comparison of ultrasound, computed tomography, and combined ultrasound with computed tomography. American Thyroid Association. 2008;**18**(4):411-418

[40] Suh CH, Baek JH, Choi YJ, Lee JH. Performance of CT in the preoperative diagnosis of cervical lymph node

metastasis in patients with papillary thyroid cancer: A systematic review and meta-analysis. AJNR. American Journal of Neuroradiology. 2017;**38**(1):154-161

[41] Yeh MW, Bauer AJ, Bernet VA, Ferris RL, Loevner LA, Mandel SJ, et al. American thyroid association statement on preoperative imaging for thyroid cancer surgery. Thyroid. 2015;**25**(1):3-14

[42] Robbins RJ, Wan Q, Grewal RK, Reibke R, Gonen M, Strauss HW, et al. Real-time prognosis for metastatic thyroid carcinoma based on 2-[18F] Fluoro-2-Deoxy-d-glucose-positron emission tomography scanning. The Journal of Clinical Endocrinology and Metabolism. 2006;**91**(2):498-505

[43] Wang W, Macapinlac H, Larson SM, Yeh SDJ, Akhurst T, Finn RD, et al. [18F]-2-Fluoro-2-Deoxy-d-glucose positron emission tomography localizes residual thyroid cancer in patients with negative diagnostic 131I whole body scans and elevated serum thyroglobulin levels. The Journal of Clinical Endocrinology and Metabolism. 1999;**84**(7):2291-2302

[44] Grünwald F, Kälicke T, Feine U, Lietzenmayer R, Scheidhauer K, Dietlein M, et al. Fluorine-18 fluorodeoxyglucose positron emission tomography in thyroid cancer: Results of a multicentre study. European Journal of Nuclear Medicine. 1999;**26**(12):1547-1552

[45] Jeong HS, Baek CH, Son YI, Choi JY, Kim HJ, Ko YH, et al. Integrated 18F-FDG PET/CT for the initial evaluation of cervical node level of patients with papillary thyroid carcinoma: Comparison with ultrasound and contrast-enhanced CT. Clinical Endocrinology. 2006;**65**(3):402-407

[46] Kim K, Shim SR, Lee SW, Kim SJ. Diagnostic values of F-18 FDG PET or PET/CT, CT, and US for preoperative lymph node staging in thyroid cancer: A network meta-analysis. The British Journal of Radiology. 2021;**94**(1120):20201076

[47] Noguchi S, Murakami N, Yamashita H, Toda M, Kawamoto H. Papillary thyroid carcinoma: Modified radical neck dissection improves prognosis. Archives of surgery (Chicago, Ill). 1998;**133**(3):276-280

[48] Scheumann GF, Gimm O, Wegener G, Hundeshagen H, Dralle H. Prognostic significance and surgical management of locoregional lymph node metastases in papillary thyroid cancer. World Journal of Surgery. 1994;**18**(4):559-567 discussion 567-568

[49] Podnos YD, Smith D, Wagman LD, Ellenhorn JDI. The implication of lymph node metastasis on survival in patients with well-differentiated thyroid cancer. The American Surgeon. 2005;**71**(9):731-734

[50] Smith VA, Sessions RB, Lentsch EJ. Cervical lymph node metastasis and papillary thyroid carcinoma: Does the compartment involved affect survival? Experience from the SEER database. Journal of Surgical Oncology. 2012;**106**(4):357-362

[51] Randolph GW, Duh QY, Heller KS, LiVolsi VA, Mandel SJ, Steward DL, et al. The prognostic significance of nodal metastases from papillary thyroid carcinoma can be stratified based on the size and number of metastatic lymph nodes, as well as the presence of extranodal extension. American Thyroid Association. 2012;**22**(11):1144-1152

[52] Schneider DF, Mazeh H, Chen H, Sippel RS. Lymph node ratio predicts recurrence in papillary thyroid cancer. The Oncologist. 2013;**18**(2):157-162

[53] Wada N, Duh QY, Sugino K, Iwasaki H, Kameyama K, Mimura T, et al. Lymph node metastasis from 259 papillary thyroid microcarcinomas: Frequency, pattern of occurrence and recurrence, and optimal strategy for neck dissection. Annals of Surgery. 2003;**237**(3):399-407

[54] Ito Y, Tomoda C, Uruno T, Takamura Y, Miya A, Kobayashi K, et al. Preoperative ultrasonographic examination for lymph node metastasis: Usefulness when designing lymph node dissection for papillary microcarcinoma of the thyroid. World Journal of Surgery. 2004;**28**(5):498-501

[55] Wada N, Suganuma N, Nakayama H, Masudo K, Rino Y, Masuda M, et al. Microscopic regional lymph node status in papillary thyroid carcinoma with and without lymphadenopathy and its relation to outcomes. Langenbeck's Archives of Surgery. 2007;**392**(4):417-422

[56] Bardet S, Malville E, Rame JP, Babin E, Samama G, De Raucourt D, et al. Macroscopic lymph-node involvement and neck dissection predict lymph-node recurrence in papillary thyroid carcinoma. European Journal of Endocrinology. 2008;**158**(4):551-560

[57] Viola D, Materazzi G, Valerio L, Molinaro E, Agate L, Faviana P, et al. Prophylactic central compartment lymph node dissection in papillary thyroid carcinoma: Clinical implications derived from the first prospective randomized controlled single institution study. The Journal of Clinical Endocrinology and Metabolism. 2015;**100**(4):1316-1324

[58] AJCC Cancer Staging Manual [Internet]. 2022. Available from: https://link.springer.com/book/9780387884400

[59] Haugen BR, Alexander EK, Bible KC, Doherty GM, Mandel SJ, Nikiforov YE, et al. 2015 American thyroid association management guidelines for adult patients with thyroid nodules and differentiated thyroid cancer: The American thyroid association guidelines task force on thyroid nodules and differentiated thyroid cancer. Thyroid. 2016;**26**(1):1-133

[60] Musacchio MJ, Kim AW, Vijungco JD, Prinz RA. Greater local recurrence occurs with 'berry picking' than neck dissection in thyroid cancer. The American Surgeon. 2003;**69**(3):191-196. discussion 196-197

[61] Sippel RS, Chen H. Controversies in the surgical management of newly diagnosed and recurrent/residual thyroid cancer. American Thyroid Association. 2009;**19**(12):1373-1380

[62] Chisholm EJ, Kulinskaya E, Tolley NS. Systematic review and meta-analysis of the adverse effects of thyroidectomy combined with central neck dissection as compared with thyroidectomy alone. The Laryngoscope. 2009;**119**(6):1135-1139

[63] Cheah WK, Arici C, Ituarte PHG, Siperstein AE, Duh QY, Clark OH. Complications of neck dissection for thyroid cancer. World Journal of Surgery. 2002;**26**(8):1013-1016

[64] Toniato A, Boschin IM, Piotto A, Pelizzo MR, Guolo A, Foletto M, et al. Complications in thyroid surgery for carcinoma: One institution's surgical experience. World Journal of Surgery. 2008;**32**(4):572-575

[65] Giordano D, Valcavi R, Thompson GB, Pedroni C, Renna L, Gradoni P, et al. Complications of central neck dissection in patients with papillary thyroid carcinoma: Results of a study on 1087 patients and review of the literature. American Thyroid Association. 2012;**22**(9):911-917

[66] Kupferman ME, Weinstock YE, Santillan AA, Mishra A, Roberts D, Clayman GL, et al. Predictors of level V metastasis in well-differentiated thyroid cancer. Head & Neck. 2008;**30**(11):1469-1474

[67] Merdad M, Eskander A, Kroeker T, Freeman JL. Metastatic papillary thyroid cancer with lateral neck disease: Pattern of spread by level. Head & Neck. 2013;**35**(10):1439-1442

[68] Farrag T, Lin F, Brownlee N, Kim M, Sheth S, Tufano RP. Is routine dissection of level II-B and V-A necessary in patients with papillary thyroid cancer undergoing lateral neck dissection for FNA-confirmed metastases in other levels. World Journal of Surgery. 2009;**33**(8):1680-1683

[69] Lee J, Sung TY, Nam KH, Chung WY, Soh EY, Park CS. Is level IIb lymph node dissection always necessary in N1b papillary thyroid carcinoma patients? World Journal of Surgery. 2008;**32**(5):716-721

[70] Patel KN, Yip L, Lubitz CC, Grubbs EG, Miller BS, Shen W, et al. The American association of endocrine surgeons guidelines for the definitive surgical management of thyroid disease in adults. Annals of Surgery. 2020;**271**(3):E21-E93

[71] Garau LM, Rubello D, Ferretti A, Boni G, Volterrani D, Manca G. Sentinel lymph node biopsy in small papillary thyroid cancer. A review on novel surgical techniques. Endocrine. 2018;**62**(2):340-350

[72] Garau LM, Rubello D, Morganti R, Boni G, Volterrani D, Colletti PM, et al. Sentinel lymph node biopsy in small papillary thyroid cancer: A meta-analysis. Clinical Nuclear Medicine. 2019;**44**(2):107-118

[73] González O, Iglesias C, Zafon C, Castellví J, García-Burillo A, Temprana J, et al. Detection of thyroid papillary carcinoma lymph node metastases using one step nucleic acid amplification (OSNA): Preliminary results. Journal of Investigative Surgery. 2015;**28**(3):153-159

[74] Amir A, Payne R, Richardson K, Hier M, Mlynarek A, Caglar D. Sentinel lymph node biopsy in thyroid cancer: It can work but there are pitfalls. Otolaryngology–Head and Neck Surgery. 2011;**145**(5):723-726

[75] Balasubramanian SP, Brignall J, Lin HY, Stephenson TJ, Wadsley J, Harrison BJ, et al. Sentinel node biopsy in papillary thyroid cancer—what is the potential? Langenbeck's Archives of Surgery. 2014;**399**(2):245-251

[76] Mazzaferri EL, Jhiang SM. Long-term impact of initial surgical and medical therapy on papillary and follicular thyroid cancer. The American Journal of Medicine. 1994;**97**(5):418-428

[77] Vaisman F, Tala H, Grewal R, Tuttle RM. In differentiated thyroid cancer, an incomplete structural response to therapy is associated with significantly worse clinical outcomes than only an incomplete thyroglobulin response. American Thyroid Association. 2011;**21**(12):1317-1322

[78] Robenshtok E, Fish S, Bach A, Domínguez JM, Shaha A, Tuttle RM. Suspicious cervical lymph nodes detected after thyroidectomy for papillary thyroid cancer usually remain stable over years in properly selected patients. The Journal of Clinical Endocrinology and Metabolism. 2012;**97**(8):2706-2713

[79] Ito Y, Higashiyama T, Takamura Y, Kobayashi K, Miya A, Miyauchi A. Prognosis of patients with papillary

thyroid carcinoma showing postoperative recurrence to the central neck. World Journal of Surgery. 2011;**35**(4):767-772

[80] Steward DL. Update in utility of secondary node dissection for papillary thyroid cancer. The Journal of Clinical Endocrinology and Metabolism. 2012;**97**(10):3393-3398

[81] Tufano RP, Clayman G, Heller KS, Inabnet WB, Kebebew E, Shaha A, et al. Management of recurrent/persistent nodal disease in patients with differentiated thyroid cancer: A critical review of the risks and benefits of surgical intervention versus active surveillance. Thyroid. 2015;**25**(1):15-27

[82] Lang BHH, Shek TWH, Chan AOK, Lo CY, Wan KY. Significance of size of persistent/recurrent central nodal disease on surgical morbidity and response to therapy in reoperative neck dissection for papillary thyroid carcinoma. Thyroid. 2017;**27**(1):67-73

[83] Rosenthal MS, Angelos P, Cooper DS, Fassler C, Finder SG, Hays MT, et al. Clinical and professional ethics guidelines for the practice of thyroidology. American Thyroid Association. 2013;**23**(10):1203-1210

[84] Sabra MM, Grewal RK, Tala H, Larson SM, Tuttle RM. Clinical outcomes following empiric radioiodine therapy in patients with structurally identifiable metastatic follicular cell-derived thyroid carcinoma with negative diagnostic but positive post-therapy 131I whole-body scans. American Thyroid Association. 2012;**22**(9):877-883

[85] Lewis BD, Hay ID, Charboneau JW, McIver B, Reading CC, Goellner JR. Percutaneous ethanol injection for treatment of cervical lymph node metastases in patients with papillary thyroid carcinoma. AJR. American Journal of Roentgenology. 2002;**178**(3):699-704

[86] Heilo A, Sigstad E, Fagerlid KH, Håskjold OI, Grøholt KK, Berner A, et al. Efficacy of ultrasound-guided percutaneous ethanol injection treatment in patients with a limited number of metastatic cervical lymph nodes from papillary thyroid carcinoma. The Journal of Clinical Endocrinology and Metabolism. 2011;**96**(9):2750-2755

[87] Hay ID, Lee RA, Davidge-Pitts C, Reading CC, Charboneau JW. Long-term outcome of ultrasound-guided percutaneous ethanol ablation of selected 'recurrent' neck nodal metastases in 25 patients with TNM stages III or IVA papillary thyroid carcinoma previously treated by surgery and 131I therapy. Surgery. 2013;**154**(6):1448-1454. discussion 1454-1455

[88] Baek JH, Kim YS, Sung JY, Choi H, Lee JH. Locoregional control of metastatic well-differentiated thyroid cancer by ultrasound-guided radiofrequency ablation. AJR. American Journal of Roentgenology. 2011;**197**(2):W331-W336

[89] Ballantyne AJ. Resections of the upper aerodigestive tract for locally invasive thyroid cancer. American Journal of Surgery. 1994;**168**(6):636-639

[90] Perros P, Boelaert K, Colley S, Evans C, Evans RM, Gerrard Ba G, et al. Guidelines for the management of thyroid cancer. Clinical Endocrinology. 2014;**81**(Suppl. 1):1-122

[91] Romesser PB, Sherman EJ, Shaha AR, Lian M, Wong RJ, Sabra M, et al. External beam radiotherapy with or without concurrent chemotherapy in advanced or recurrent non-anaplastic non-medullary thyroid cancer. Journal of Surgical Oncology. 2014;**110**(4):375-382

[92] Rothenberg SM, McFadden DG, Palmer EL, Daniels GH, Wirth LJ. Redifferentiation of iodine-refractory BRAF V600E-mutant metastatic papillary thyroid cancer with dabrafenib. Clinical Cancer Research. 2015;**21**(5):1028-1035

Chapter 10

External Beam Radiotherapy in Differentiated Thyroid Cancer

Lekha Madhavan Nair, Rejnish Ravikumar, Malu Rafi, Mullangath Prakasan Aparna, Zuzaki Sharafuddin, John Mohan Mathew and Kainickal Cessal Thommachan

Abstract

Differentiated thyroid cancer is treated by surgery, radioiodine treatment, and Thyroid Stimulating Hormone (TSH) suppression. The role of external beam radiotherapy is mainly palliation of radio-iodine non avid metastatic lesions and in inoperable tumors. Metastasis involving weight-bearing bones and vertebral metastasis with impending spinal cord compression are primarily treated by external radiation. External Beam Radiotherapy improves loco-regional control in patients with gross residual disease after surgical resection. Patients with extra-thyroidal disease and positive margins are treated by adjuvant external beam radiotherapy, especially when the post op radio-iodine scan is negative. External beam radiotherapy is the treatment of choice for radio-iodine non avid inoperable loco-regional recurrence. SRS alone or surgery followed by SRS is the preferred treatment for solitary brain metastasis. Whole brain radiotherapy is the treatment of choice for multiple brain metastatic disease.

Keywords: differentiated thyroid cancer, external beam radiotherapy, iodine refractory disease, thyroid stimulating hormone (TSH), metastatic disease

1. Introduction

Differentiated thyroid cancer (DTC) is treated by surgery, thyroid stimulating hormone (TSH) suppression, and radioiodine therapy according to the risk stratification [1, 2]. External Beam Radiotherapy (EBRT) is used in selected patients in the adjuvant setting. EBRT is mainly used in the palliation of radio-iodine non-avid metastatic disease and inoperable tumors. There are no prospective randomized trials on EBRT in DTC. The available evidence is from single institution retrospective studies, systematic reviews, and meta-analysis. In this chapter, we discuss the role of EBRT in localized and metastatic DTC. **Figure 1** summarizes the role of EBRT in differentiated thyroid cancer.

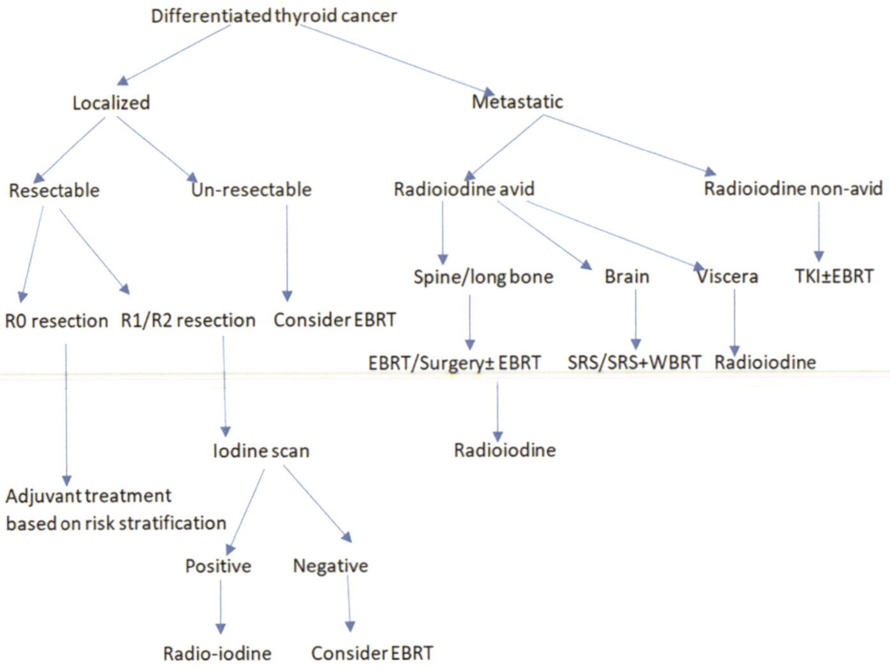

Figure 1.
The role of EBRT in differentiated thyroid cancer.

2. Localized disease

2.1 Gross loco-regional residual disease after surgery

The definition of gross residual disease is not clearly defined in the published literature. EBRT improves loco-regional control in patients with gross residual disease after surgical resection. Most of the retrospective studies utilized radio-iodine in addition to EBRT. Hence the magnitude of benefit from EBRT alone is not known. In patients less than 55 years old with limited radio-iodine avid gross residual disease, EBRT is not indicated as radio-iodine alone may be sufficient for local control. In patients with radio-iodine concentrating residual disease, radio-iodine treatment is considered first and EBRT is given after radio-iodine to avoid the stunning effect of EBRT. EBRT is considered before radioiodine treatment in cases where the residual disease is likely to compromise the airway.

In a retrospective study from Queen Elizabeth hospital China with 842 patients, EBRT was effective in increasing local control in patients with gross residual disease [3]. At Memorial Sloan Kettering Cancer Center, 2 and 4 year loco-regional control with EBRT was 77% and 62%, respectively, for patients with gross residual disease [4]. Meadows et al. reported 5 year local control rate of 70% for patients with gross residual disease [5]. In a retrospective study, Sia et al. reported 10 year local relapse free rate of 90% with EBRT for those with gross residual disease [6]. Beckham et al. have reported the outcome of DTC patients treated with IMRT and concurrent Doxorubicin in patients with un-resectable and gross residual disease. Patients who received concurrent chemotherapy had better local progression-free survival and overall survival than those who received only IMRT [7]. EBRT is primarily considered for macroscopic residual disease in case of radio-iodine non avid residual disease. EBRT may be considered after radio-iodine treatment if the residual disease is unlikely to be controlled with radio-iodine treatment alone.

2.2 T4 disease after complete surgical resection or microscopic margin positivity

Radio-iodine is the treatment of choice for extra-thyroidal extension and microscopic positive margins. EBRT is not routinely recommended in this scenario. EBRT may be recommended in patients with microscopic residual disease and aggressive histological subtypes which are unlikely to concentrate iodine.

A randomized control trial was designed in Germany with pT4 patients in the EBRT arm and no EBRT arm, but due to poor accrual it was converted into a prospective cohort study. The RT dose to the thyroid bed was 59.4Gy for R0 resection and 66.6Gy for R1 resection. The complete remission rate was 96% with EBRT versus 86% without EBRT, and the study concluded that EBRT could not be routinely recommended for all pT4 disease [8]. Schwartz et al. reported a loco-regional control rate of 81% after EBRT in patients with extra-thyroidal disease or microscopic positive margins [9]. The median dose was 60 Gy for negative margins or microscopic positive margins. Over a 40-year period, Princess Margaret Hospital experience demonstrated benefit in LRC with EBRT of 45–50 Gy for patients >60 years, T4 disease without gross residue [10]. Kim et al. reported improvement in LRC for T4 or node positive disease with EBRT doses of 50–70 Gy [11]. The role of EBRT in patients with tracheal invasion was reported by Keum et al. and Kim et al. in 2 separate publications. Both these studies reported superior loco-regional control with EBRT [12, 13]. In another retrospective study by Groen et al., 5 year LRC was 84.3% with EBRT (66 Gy) for microscopic residual disease [14].

EBRT may be considered for patients with extra-thyroidal extension or microscopic positive margins that are radio-iodine non-avid.

2.3 Un-resectable DTC

Palliative EBRT is recommended to relieve symptoms in un-resectable DTC [15]. In a retrospective cohort study by Carrillo et al., un-resectable DTC patients were treated with EBRT or EBRT followed by salvage surgery. Patients with ECOG performance status≤2 received doses above 56 Gy and a palliative dose of 30–50 Gy was used for patients with poor performance status. IMRT followed by salvage surgery was associated with increased Progression Free Survival and Overall Survival [16].

2.4 Inoperable loco-regional recurrence

The most common sites of failure in DTC are the thyroid bed and regional nodes. The treatment of choice for loco-regional recurrence is salvage surgery followed by radioiodine treatment. EBRT is considered after surgery when there is extensive extra-thyroidal extension or extra-capsular spread of lymphnodes at recurrence [17]. Some patients may develop loco-regional recurrence not amenable to surgery or radio-iodine. EBRT is the preferred treatment modality in such cases [4, 18]. The dose ranges from 66 to 70 Gy.

2.5 Evidence from systematic reviews and meta-analysis

A systematic review of 16 studies by Fussy et al. reported an improvement in LRC with post-op EBRT in patients at high risk for recurrence and above 45 years of age [19]. Another systematic review and meta-analysis by Dicuonzo et al. also reported improvement in loco-regional control with the addition of EBRT to surgery and radio-iodine without considerable toxicity [20]. Jacomina et al. conducted a systematic review and meta-analysis of 9 trials and reported improvement in 5 year loco-regional recurrence free survival with post-operative EBRT in patients with advanced age, gross or microscopic residual disease, and loco-regionally advanced disease. However, there was no improvement in overall survival or distant metastasis failure-free survival [21]. A recent review by Roukoz and Gregoire concluded that adjuvant EBRT reduces the risk of loco-regional recurrence in locally advanced DTC with high-risk features [22].

2.6 Radiotherapy-Pretreatment evaluation, technique, dose, and volumes

Dental, speech, swallowing, and nutritional evaluation should be done prior to radiotherapy. Pre-treatment contrast enhanced CT, MRI, and whole body iodine scans can be used for delineation of target volumes. The target volumes should include any gross residual disease, the thyroid bed, including the trachea-esophageal grove and draining lymph nodes (peri-thyroidal lymph nodes, para-tracheal, pre-tracheal, superior mediastinum and cervical lymph nodes). PET CT helps in the delineation of gross tumors, especially in iodine refractory disease [23]. Intensity Modulated Radiotherapy (IMRT) is the technique of choice for EBRT in DTC [7, 24–26]. IMRT ensures appropriate coverage of volumes and it spares more normal tissues compared to 3 Dimensional Conformal Radiotherapy. It also allows for dose escalation without increasing toxicity [27]. The recommended EBRT dose is 66–70 Gy for gross residual or un-resectable disease, 60–66 Gy for microscopic disease, and 50–56 Gy for elective nodal regions [28, 29]. Gross residual nodes are treated with 66–70 Gy and nodes with extra-capsular extension are treated with 60–66 Gy.

2.7 Radiotherapy toxicities

Acute toxicities of radiotherapy include skin erythema, desquamation, mucositis, and dysphagia. Esophageal and tracheal stenosis, chronic dysphagia, feeding tube dependency, and xerostomia are the late side effects. According to the study by Schuck et al., acute grade 3 toxicity in the larynx, pharynx, and skin of any grade was reported in only 9.1% of patients and there were no late grade 3 toxicities after EBRT [30].

3. Metastatic disease

The EBRT is used for symptomatic metastatic disease that is not amenable to surgery or radio-iodine. The most common sites of metastases from DTC are bone and lungs. Radio-iodine-avid metastatic bone lesions are treated by radio-iodine. Palliative surgery is recommended for patients who have a pathological fracture or spinal cord compression and a limited volume of metastatic disease. EBRT is used to complement surgery in such situations [31]. EBRT is primarily considered in cases of metastases involving weight-bearing bones and vertebrae with impending spinal cord compression [32]. Stereotactic radiosurgery is effective for oligo-metastatic bone lesions [33–35]. Due to prolonged survival in DTC, hypo fractionated regimens like 40 Gy in 15 fractions or 30 Gy in 10 fractions are recommended. Less protracted regimens like 20 Gy in 5 fractions or 8 Gy single fraction EBRT can be considered in patients with disseminated metastatic disease [36]. Multiple cerebral metastases are usually treated by whole brain RT (30 Gy in 10 fractions or 20 Gy in 5 fractions) as radio-iodine is likely to aggravate cerebral edema [37]. Solitary brain metastasis is treated by surgical excision or stereotactic radiosurgery (SRS). Surgical excision followed by SRS or SRS alone can be considered for ≤4 brain metastases [36]. SRS is reported to be safe in patients with DTC and it results in durable intracranial disease control [38]. The systemic treatment of choice for iodine refractory metastatic differentiated thyroid cancer is tyrosine kinase inhibitors (TKI). Sorafenib and Lenvatinib are approved for the treatment of iodine refractory disease in the first line setting [39, 40]. Cabozantinib is approved for patients previously treated with vascular endothelial growth factor receptor (VEGFR)-targeted therapy [41]. At present, there is no concrete data to alter the indication for palliative radiotherapy in metastatic disease in the TKI era.

4. Future directions

EBRT is the treatment of choice for iodine refractory DTC recurrence. A pilot study conducted on F18 FDG PET guided EBRT showed promising results [42]. PETCT identifies relapsed sites and allows dose escalation to sites of recurrence. It helps in reducing treatment volumes, thereby reducing adverse effects. Initial experience on Intensity Modulated Proton Therapy (IMPT) from Mayo Clinic has been published and showed promising loco-regional control for recurrent iodine refractory DTC [43, 44]. The long term efficacy and safety of proton beam therapy are yet to be proven.

5. Conclusions

EBRT reduces the risk of loco-regional recurrence in locally advanced DTC. EBRT is indicated in gross loco-regional residual disease after surgery, extra-thyroidal extension with radioiodine non avid microscopic residual disease, inoperable loco-regional recurrence which fails to concentrate iodine; and in the palliation of metastatic disease.

Author details

Lekha Madhavan Nair, Rejnish Ravikumar, Malu Rafi, Mullangath Prakasan Aparna, Zuzaki Sharafuddin, John Mohan Mathew and Kainickal Cessal Thommachan*
Department of Radiation Oncology, Regional Cancer Centre, Thiruvananthapuram, Kerala, India

*Address all correspondence to: drcessalthomas@gmail.com

References

[1] Haugen BR, Alexander EK, Bible KC, Doherty GM, Mandel SJ, Nikiforov YE, et al. 2015 American Thyroid Association management guidelines for adult patients with thyroid nodules and differentiated thyroid Cancer: The American Thyroid Association guidelines task force on thyroid nodules and differentiated thyroid Cancer. Thyroid Official Journal of American Thyroid Association. 2016;**26**(1):1-133

[2] Filetti S, Durante C, Hartl D, Leboulleux S, Locati LD, Newbold K, et al. Thyroid cancer: ESMO clinical practice guidelines for diagnosis, treatment and follow-up. Annals of Oncology. 2019;**30**(12):1856-1883

[3] Chow SM, Law SCK, Mendenhall WM, Au SK, Chan PTM, Leung TW, et al. Papillary thyroid carcinoma: Prognostic factors and the role of radioiodine and external radiotherapy. International Journal of Radiation Oncology. 2002;**52**(3):784-795

[4] Terezakis SA, Lee KS, Ghossein RA, Rivera M, Tuttle RM, Wolden SL, et al. Role of external beam radiotherapy in patients with advanced or recurrent nonanaplastic thyroid cancer: Memorial Sloan-Kettering Cancer Center experience. International Journal of Radiation Oncology, Biology, Physics. 2009;**73**(3):795-801

[5] Meadows KM, Amdur RJ, Morris CG, Villaret DB, Mazzaferri EL, Mendenhall WM. External beam radiotherapy for differentiated thyroid cancer. American Journal of Otolaryngology. 2006;**27**(1):24-28

[6] Sia MA, Tsang RW, Panzarella T, Brierley JD. Differentiated thyroid Cancer with extrathyroidal extension: Prognosis and the role of external beam radiotherapy. Journal of Thyroid Research. 2010;**2010**:1-7

[7] Beckham TH, Romesser PB, Groen AH, Sabol C, Shaha AR, Sabra M, et al. Intensity-modulated radiation therapy with or without concurrent chemotherapy in nonanaplastic thyroid Cancer with unresectable or gross residual disease. Thyroid Official Journal of American Thyroid Association. 2018;**28**(9):1180-1189

[8] Biermann M, Pixberg M, Riemann B, Schuck A, Heinecke A, Schmid KW, et al. Clinical outcomes of adjuvant external-beam radiotherapy for differentiated thyroid cancer - results after 874 patient-years of follow-up in the MSDS-trial. Nuclear Medicine. 2009;**48**(3):89-98

[9] Schwartz DL, Lobo MJ, Ang KK, Morrison WH, Rosenthal DI, Ahamad A, et al. Postoperative external beam radiotherapy for differentiated thyroid Cancer: Outcomes and morbidity with conformal treatment. International Journal of Radiation Oncology. 2009;**74**(4):1083-1091

[10] Brierley J, Tsang R, Panzarella T, Bana N. Prognostic factors and the effect of treatment with radioactive iodine and external beam radiation on patients with differentiated thyroid cancer seen at a single institution over 40 years. Clinical Endocrinology. 2005;**63**(4):418-427

[11] Kim TH, Yang DS, Jung KY, Kim CY, Choi MS. Value of external irradiation for locally advanced papillary thyroid cancer. International Journal of Radiation Oncology. 2003;**55**(4):1006-1012

[12] Keum KC, Suh YG, Koom WS, Cho JH, Shim SJ, Lee CG, et al. The role of postoperative external-beam

radiotherapy in the management of patients with papillary thyroid cancer invading the trachea. International Journal of Radiation Oncology, Biology, Physics. 2006;**65**(2):474-480

[13] Kim YS, Choi JH, Kim KS, Lim GC, Kim JH, Kang JW, et al. The role of adjuvant external beam radiation therapy for papillary thyroid carcinoma invading the trachea. Radiation Oncology Journal. 2017;**35**(2):112-120

[14] Groen AH, van Dijk D, Sluiter W, et al. Postoperative external beam radiotherapy for locoregional control in iodine refractory differentiated thyroid cancer. European Thyroid Journal. Jan 2022;**11**(1):e210033. DOI: 10.1530/etj-21-0033. PMID: 34981752; PMCID: PMC9142801

[15] Mitchell AL, Gandhi A, Scott-Coombes D, Perros P. Management of thyroid cancer: United Kingdom National Multidisciplinary Guidelines. The Journal of Laryngology and Otology. 2016;**130**(S2):S150-S160

[16] Carrillo JF, Flores JM, Espinoza G, Vázquez-Romo R, Ramírez-Ortega MC, Carrillo LC, et al. Treatment of unresectable differentiated thyroid carcinoma with upfront external radiotherapy and salvage surgery: A STROBE-compliant retrospective cohort study. Frontiers in Oncology. 2021;**10**:572958

[17] Lee N, Tuttle M. The role of external beam radiotherapy in the treatment of papillary thyroid cancer. Endocrine-Related Cancer. 2006;**13**(4):971-977

[18] Romesser PB, Sherman EJ, Shaha AR, Lian M, Wong RJ, Sabra M, et al. External beam radiotherapy with or without concurrent chemotherapy in advanced or recurrent non-anaplastic non-medullary thyroid cancer: EBRT in advanced or recurrent thyroid Cancer. Journal of Surgical Oncology. 2014;**110**(4):375-382

[19] Fussey JM, Crunkhorn R, Tedla M, Weickert MO, Mehanna H. External beam radiotherapy in differentiated thyroid carcinoma: A systematic review: External beam radiotherapy in differentiated thyroid carcinoma. Eisele DW, editor. Head & Neck. 2016;**38**(S1):E2297-E2305

[20] Dicuonzo S, Pedretti S, Mangoni M, Monari F, Fanetti G, Borsatti E, et al. Adjuvant radiotherapy and radioiodine treatment for locally advanced differentiated thyroid cancer: Systematic review and meta-analysis. Tumori Journal. 2021;**107**(6):489-497

[21] Jacomina LE, Jacinto JKM, Co LBA, Yu KKL, Agas RAF, Co JL, et al. The role of postoperative external beam radiotherapy for differentiated thyroid carcinoma: A systematic review and meta-analysis. Head & Neck. 2020;**42**(8):2181-2193

[22] Roukoz C, Gregoire V. Indications of external beams radiation for thyroid cancer. Current Opinion in Otolaryngology & Head and Neck Surgery. 2022;**30**(2):137-144

[23] Marcus C, Whitworth PW, Surasi DS, Pai SI, Subramaniam RM. PET/CT in the management of thyroid cancers. AJR. American Journal of Roentgenology. 2014;**202**(6):1316-1329

[24] Nutting CM, Convery DJ, Cosgrove VP, Rowbottom C, Vini L, Harmer C, et al. Improvements in target coverage and reduced spinal cord irradiation using intensity-modulated radiotherapy (IMRT) in patients with carcinoma of the thyroid gland. Radiotherapy Oncology Journal of European Society. 2001;**60**(2):173-180

[25] Rosenbluth BD, Serrano V, Happersett L, Shaha AR, Tuttle RM, Narayana A, et al. Intensity-modulated radiation therapy for the treatment of nonanaplastic thyroid cancer. International Journal of Radiation Oncology, Biology, Physics. 2005;**63**(5): 1419-1426

[26] Sun XS, Sun SR, Guevara N, Marcy PY, Peyrottes I, Lassalle S, et al. Indications of external beam radiation therapy in non-anaplastic thyroid cancer and impact of innovative radiation techniques. Critical Reviews in Oncology/Hematology. 2013;**86**(1):52-68

[27] Brierley JD. Update on external beam radiation therapy in thyroid Cancer. The Journal of Clinical Endocrinology and Metabolism. 2011;**96**(8):2289-2295

[28] Perros P, Boelaert K, Colley S, Evans C, Evans RM, Gerrard BAG, et al. Guidelines for the management of thyroid cancer. Clinical Endocrinology. 2014;**81**:1-122

[29] Kiess AP, Agrawal N, Brierley JD, Duvvuri U, Ferris RL, Genden E, et al. External-beam radiotherapy for differentiated thyroid cancer locoregional control: A statement of the American head and neck society: External-beam RT for differentiated thyroid cancer. Head & Neck. 2016;**38**(4):493-498

[30] Schuck A, Biermann M, Pixberg MK, Müller SB, Heinecke A, Schober O, et al. Acute toxicity of adjuvant radiotherapy in locally advanced differentiated thyroid carcinoma. First results of the multicenter study differentiated thyroid carcinoma (MSDS). Strahlenther Onkol Organ Dtsch Rontgengesellschaft Al. 2003;**179**(12):832-839

[31] Kato S, Demura S, Shinmura K, Yokogawa N, Shimizu T, Tsuchiya H. Current Management of Bone Metastases from differentiated thyroid Cancer. Cancers. 2021;**13**(17):4429

[32] Filetti S, Durante C, Hartl DM, Leboulleux S, Locati LD, Newbold K, et al. ESMO clinical practice guideline update on the use of systemic therapy in advanced thyroid cancer. Annals of Oncology. 2022

[33] Ishigaki T, Uruno T, Sugino K, Masaki C, Akaishi J, Hames KY, et al. Stereotactic radiotherapy using the CyberKnife is effective for local control of bone metastases from differentiated thyroid cancer. Journal of Radiation Research (Tokyo). 2019;**60**(6):831-836

[34] Bernstein MB, Chang EL, Amini B, Pan H, Cabanillas M, Wang XA, et al. Spine stereotactic radiosurgery for patients with metastatic thyroid Cancer: Secondary analysis of phase I/II trials. Thyroid Official Journal of American Thyroid Association. 2016;**26**(9):1269-1275

[35] Boyce-Fappiano D, Gjyshi O, Pezzi TA, Allen PK, Solimman M, Taku N, et al. Spine stereotactic radiosurgery for metastatic thyroid cancer: A single-institution experience. Journal of Neurosurgery. Spine. 2020;**14**:1-9

[36] Haddad RI, Nasr C, Bischoff L, Busaidy NL, Byrd D, Callender G, et al. NCCN guidelines insights: Thyroid carcinoma, version 2.2018. Journal of National Comprehensive Cancer Network JNCCN. 2018;**16**(12):1429-1440

[37] Tumino D, Frasca F, Newbold K. Updates on the Management of Advanced, metastatic, and radioiodine refractory differentiated thyroid Cancer. Frontiers in Endocrinology. 2017;**8**:312

[38] Bunevicius A, Fribance S, Pikis S, Lee JYK, Buch LY, Moran M, et al. Stereotactic radiosurgery for differentiated thyroid Cancer brain

metastases: An international, Multicenter study. Thyroid Official Journal of American Thyroid Association. 2021;**31**(8):1244-1252

[39] Brose MS, Nutting CM, Jarzab B, Elisei R, Siena S, Bastholt L, et al. Sorafenib in radioactive iodine-refractory, locally advanced or metastatic differentiated thyroid cancer: A randomised, double-blind, phase 3 trial. Lancet London England. 2014;**384**(9940):319-328

[40] Schlumberger M, Tahara M, Wirth LJ, Robinson B, Brose MS, Elisei R, et al. Lenvatinib versus placebo in radioiodine-refractory thyroid cancer. The New England Journal of Medicine. 2015;**372**(7):621-630

[41] Brose MS, Robinson B, Sherman SI, Krajewska J, Lin CC, Vaisman F, et al. Cabozantinib for radioiodine-refractory differentiated thyroid cancer (COSMIC-311): A randomised, double-blind, placebo-controlled, phase 3 trial. The Lancet Oncology. 2021;**22**(8):1126-1138

[42] Farina E, Monari F, Castellucci P, Romani F, Repaci A, Farina A, et al. ^{18}F-FDG pet-guided external beam radiotherapy in iodine-refractory differentiated thyroid Cancer: A pilot study. Journal of Thyroid Research. 2017;**2017**:1-9

[43] Yu NY, Khurana A, Ma DJ, Neben-Wittich MA, Golafshar MA, McGee LA, et al. Initial experience with proton beam therapy for differentiated thyroid cancer. International Journal of Part Therapy. 2021;**8**(1):311-318

[44] Yu N, Khurana A, Foote R, Ma D, Neben-Wittich M, McGee L, et al. Proton beam therapy for differentiated thyroid cancer: Initial report of the Mayo Clinic experience. International Journal of Radiation Oncology. 2020;**108**(2):E47